5 Ingredient R
Cookbo

Quick, Easy and Delicious Recipes with Low Sodium, Potassium, and Phosphorus to Manage Every Stage of Kidney Disease

Written By

Delilah Hooper

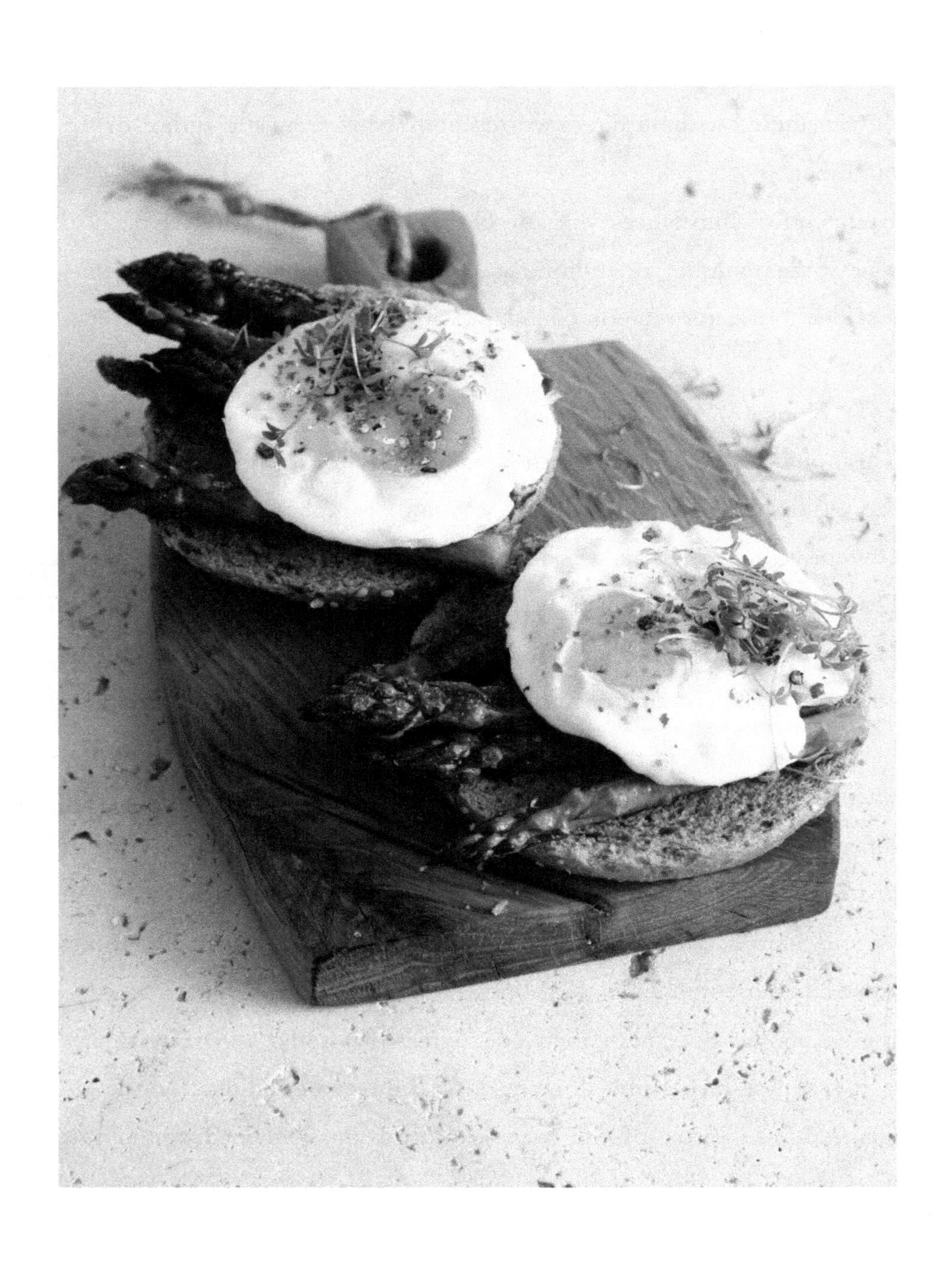

Table of Contents

Introduction

Despite their tiny size, the kidneys perform a number of functions which are vital for the body to be able to function healthily.

These include:

- Filtering excess fluids and waste from the blood
- Creating the enzyme known as renin which regulates blood pressure
- Ensuring bone marrow creates red blood cells
- Controlling calcium and phosphorus levels through absorption and excretion

Unfortunately, when kidney disease reaches a chronic stage, these functions start to stop working. However, with the right treatment and lifestyle, it is possible to manage symptoms and continue living well. This is even more applicable in the earlier stages of the disease. Tactlessly, 10% of all adults over the age of 20 will experience some form of kidney disease in their lifetime. There are a variety of different treatments for kidney disease, which depend on the cause of the disease.

Possible causes are outlined below:

- DIABETES: In the United States and other countries where the 'Standard American Diet' runs rampant, the number one leading cause of kidney disease is high blood pressure and Type 2 diabetes. Both of these diseases are either completely preventable or at least treatable and once the root issue has been treated, kidney disease issues can also dissipate.

- GLOMERULONEPHRITIS: Damage to the glomeruli (the filters in your kidneys), impairs the kidneys' ability to filter waste materials. This can be caused by damage to the immune system and if this is the case, can be treated with medication. It is either experienced for a short period of time (acute glomerulonephritis), or for a longer period of time (chronic). In chronic cases, further problems can arise such as high blood pressure, organ damage and later chronic kidney disease.
- ACUTE RENAL FAILURE/ACUTE KIDNEY INJURY:

Sudden damage or failure of the kidney can be caused by a rapid loss of blood to the kidneys, sepsis or even severe dehydration. Infection, poison and some medicines are also known to lead to acute kidney issues.

- SUDDEN BLOCKAGE: Kidney stones, tumors, injuries and an enlarged prostate in men can stop urine from passing through the kidneys as it should. This can cause swelling in the lower extremities, a loss of appetite, vomiting or nausea, extreme tiredness, restlessness, feelings of confusion, or even an acute pain beneath the ribs (known as flank pain).

- ECLAMPSIA: This can be experienced during pregnancy when the placenta doesn't function as it should do, creating high blood pressure and sometimes leading to kidney problems.

- BREAKDOWN OF MUSCLE TISSUE: Under extreme pressure, for example when running a marathon or undergoing other feats of massive exertion, the body starts to break down muscle tissue after it has used all other available fuel. If this continues unchecked, too much of the protein known as myoglobin will ultimately end up in the bloodstream, putting undue strain on the kidneys and potentially leading to further implications.

- IMMUNE SYSTEM: Common immune system diseases that can lead to kidney issues include lupus, hepatitis C, hepatitis B, HIV, and aids. These can lead to what is known as chronic kidney disease (any form of kidney disease that lasts for three months or longer). Sometimes the sufferer of the immune disease will not experience the symptoms of the kidney disease until it reaches a chronic stage; this can be dangerous as it is a lot harder to manage once it has reached this level.

- EXTREME URINARY TRACT INFECTIONS: Urinary tract infections that occur within the kidneys rather than the bladder are known as pyelonephritis and occur when a traditional urinary tract infection remains untreated long enough for it to spread into the upper urinary tract system. This can cause scarring in the kidneys which can lead to severe flaws in kidney functioning.

- STREPTOCOCCAL INFECTIONS: Commonly known as a strep infection, this bacterium can infect the throat as well as various layers of the skin, the middle ear, the sinuses or even in a more severe case, a widespread vicious rash known as scarlet fever. This bacterium is known to result in the glomeruli (individual filters in the kidneys) becoming infected.

- POLYCYSTIC KIDNEY DISEASE: This type of kidney disease is typically passed down from parent to child and causes cysts filled with fluid to form on the kidneys themselves.

- BIRTH DEFECTS: Depending on the severity of the defect, kidney disease could form simply because the kidneys do not function correctly or because of an obstruction in the urinary tract before birth.

Breakfast Recipes

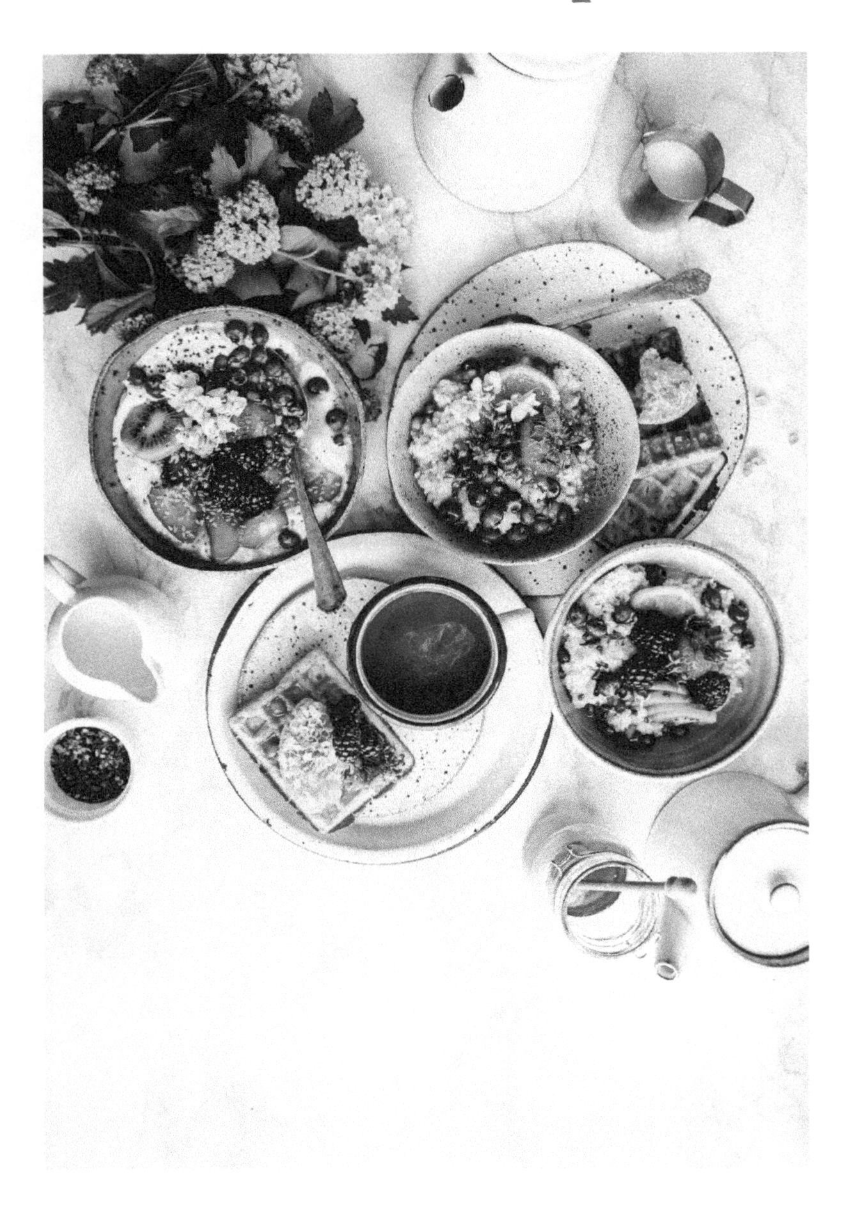

1. Strawberry Topped Waffles

Preparation Time: *15 minutes* | ***Cooking Time:*** *20 minutes* | ***Servings:*** *5*

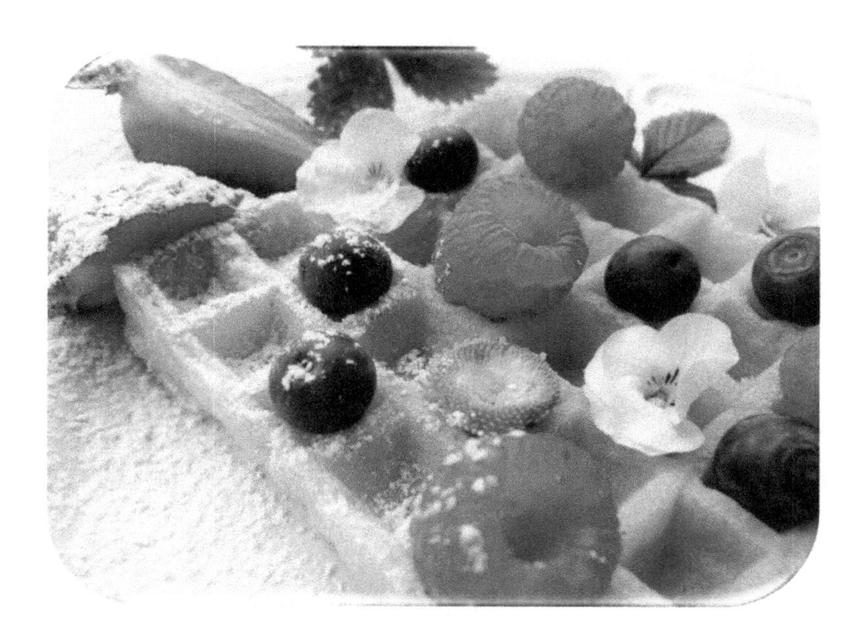

Ingredients:

- 1 cup flour
- 1/4 cup Swerve
- 1 ¾ teaspoons baking powder
- 1 egg, separated
- ¾ cup milk
- ½ cup butter, melted
- ½ teaspoon vanilla extract
- Fresh strawberries, sliced

Directions:

Prepare and preheat your waffle pan following the instructions of the machine.

Begin by mixing the flour with Swerve and baking soda in a bowl. Separate the egg yolks from the egg whites, keeping them in two separate bowls. Add the milk and vanilla extract to the egg yolks.

Stir the melted butter and mix well until smooth. Now beat the egg whites with an electric beater until foamy and fluffy.

Fold this fluffy composition in the egg yolk mixture. Mix it gently until smooth, then add in the flour mixture. Stir again to make a smooth mixture.

Pour a half cup of the waffle batter in a preheated pan and cook until the waffle is done. Cook more waffles with the remaining batter.

Serve fresh with strawberries on top.

Nutrition	Calories	Fat	Carbs	Protein	Sodium	Phosphorus	Potassium
	342	20g	21g	5g	156mg	126mg	233mg

2. Simple Fluffy Sour Cream Pancakes

Preparation Time: *15 minutes* | ***Cooking Time***: *20 minutes* | ***Servings***: *4*

Ingredients:

- 1 cup milk
- 1/2 cup sour cream
- 1 egg, slightly beaten
- 2 tablespoons sugar
- 2 tablespoons butter, melted
- 1 teaspoon vanilla extract
- 1 & 1/2 cup all-purpose flour
- 2 teaspoons baking powder
- 1 teaspoon baking soda
- 1/4 teaspoon salt

Directions:

These simple and fluffy sour cream pancakes are delicious! They are easy to make and require little effort.

The secret to a fluffy pancake is to let the batter sit for about 15 minutes on the counter-top or overnight in the fridge.

Whisk together the egg, sugar, milk, sour cream, butter, and vanilla extract. Combine the flour, baking powder, baking soda, and salt in a separate bowl.

Add the flour mixture to the liquid mixture and whisk together until no large clumps remain. Let the batter sit for 15 minutes. You can even refrigerate it overnight and cook the next morning.

Heat a nonstick pan on medium/low heat. Spray with oil or melt a dab of butter in the pan. Add the butter and cook for about 2 minutes on each side.

Serve immediately. Garnish with fresh fruit or just a simple drizzle of sticky maple syrup!

Feel free to customize the recipe and add fresh fruit or nuts into the batter; I can picture how delicious it will taste with the addition of blueberries!

Nutrition	Calories	Fat	Carbs	Protein	Sodium	Phosphorus	Potassium
	125	6g	29g	15g	48mg	159mg	279mg

3. Healthy Apple Muesli

***Preparation Time**: 10 minutes* | ***Cooking Time**: 0 minutes* |

***Servings**: 1*

Ingredients:

- 1/2 cup raw quick oats
- 1 cup milk (any type, unsweetened)
- 1 tbsp. chia seeds (or flax)
- 1/4 cup grated apple
- 1/4 tsp. ground cinnamon
- Maple syrup to taste

Directions:

A nutrition-dense breakfast that will keep you full until lunch! Combine all ingredients in a bowl and serve.

	Calories	Fat	Carbs	Protein	Sodium	Phosphorus	Potassium
Nutrition	375	14g	49g	13g	108mg	159mg	297mg

4. Mexican Frittata

Preparation Time: *15 minutes* | ***Cooking Time:*** *20 minutes* |

Servings: *4*

Ingredients:

- ½ cup almond milk
- 5 large eggs
- ¼ cup onions, chopped
- ¼ cup green bell pepper, chopped

Directions:

Preheat the oven to 400° F. Using a large bowl, combine almond milk, eggs, onion, and green bell pepper.

Whisk until all ingredients are well combined.

Transfer the mixture to a baking dish. Bake for 20 minutes. Serve.

Nutrition	Calories	Fat	Carbs	Protein	Sodium	Phosphorus	Potassium
	358	11g	39g	17g	216mg	59mg	243mg

5. Olive Oil and Sesame Asparagus

***Preparation Time**: 15 minutes* | ***Cooking Time**: 20 minutes* |

***Servings**: 4*

Ingredients:

- ½ cup of water
- 2 cups asparagus, sliced
- ½ tablespoon olive oil, add more for drizzling
- 1/8 teaspoon red pepper flakes, crushed
- ½ teaspoon sesame seeds

Directions:

In a large skillet, bring water to a boil. Add in asparagus. Allow to boil for 2 minutes. Reduce the heat and cook for another 5 minutes. Drain asparagus and place on a plate. Set aside.

Meanwhile, heat the olive oil. Tip in asparagus and red pepper flakes. Saute for 3 minutes. Remove from heat. Drizzle in more olive oil and sprinkle sesame seeds before serving.

Nutrition	Calories	Fat	Carbs	Protein	Sodium	Phosphorus	Potassium
	415	7g	39g	6.3g	9mg	59mg	547mg

6. Roasted Pepper Soup

Preparation Time: *15 minutes* | ***Cooking Time***: *30 minutes* | ***Servings***: *4*

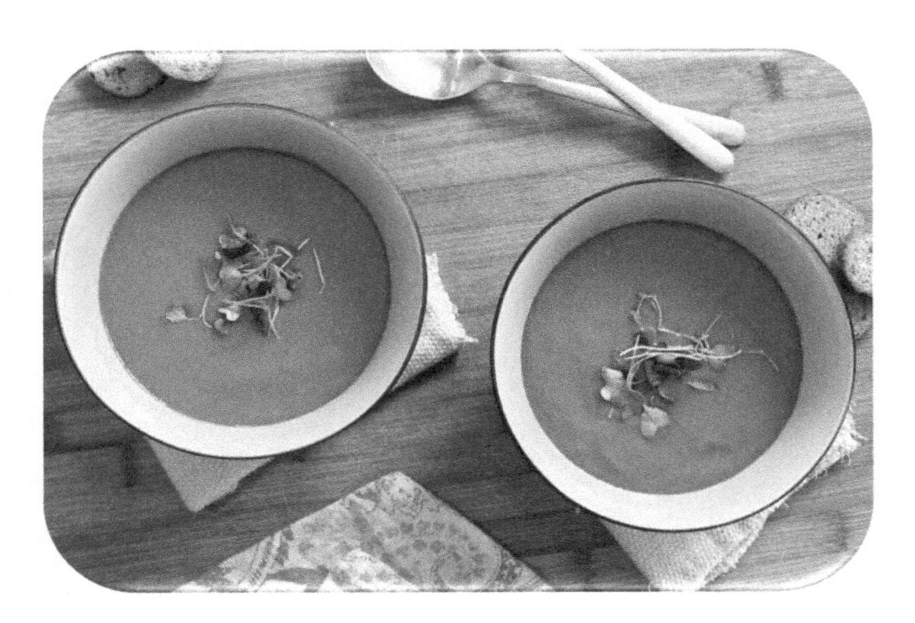

Ingredients:

- 2 tablespoons olive oil
- 2 large red peppers
- ½ cup onion, chopped
- 2 garlic cloves, minced
- ½ cup carrots, chopped
- ½ cup celery, chopped
- 2 cups vegetable broth, unsalted
- ½ cup almond milk
- ¼ cup sweet basil, julienned

Directions:

Place the oven into the 375°F. Put onions on a baking sheet. Add the red peppers beside the mixture.

Drizzle some of the olive oil over everything and toss well to coat. Roast for 20 minutes, or until peppers are tender and skins are wilted.

Chop the roasted red peppers and set aside. Place a pot over medium-high flame and heat through. Once hot, add the olive oil and swirl to coat.

Place the carrot, celery, and garlic into the pot and sauté until carrot and celery are tender. Add the chopped roasted red peppers. Mix well.

Pour in the vegetable broth and almond milk. Increase to high flame and bring to a boil. Once boiling, reduce to a simmer. Simmer, uncovered, for 10 minutes. Turn off the heat and allow to cool slightly.

If desired, blend the soup using an immersion blender until the soup has reached a desired level of smoothness.

Reheat over medium flame. Add the basil and stir to combine. Serve.

Nutrition	Calories	Fat	Carbs	Protein	Sodium	Phosphorus	Potassium
	345	4g	9g	1.3g	47mg	117mg	249mg

7. Poached Asparagus and Egg

Preparation Time: *5 minutes |* ***Cooking Time:*** *20 minutes |* ***Servings:*** *4*

Ingredients:

- 1 large egg
- 4 spears asparagus
- Water, for boiling

Directions:

Half-fill a deep saucepan with water set over high heat. Let the water come to a rolling boil. Dunk asparagus spears in water.

Cook until they turn a shade brighter, about 3 minutes. Remove from saucepan and drain on paper towels.

Keep warm. Lightly season prior to serving. Slice the top off. The egg should still be fluid inside.

To serve: place asparagus spears on a small plate and serve egg on the side. Dip asparagus into egg and eat while warm.

Nutrition	Calories	Fat	Carbs	Protein	Sodium	Phosphorus	Potassium
	245	12g	21g	7.5g	71mg	59mg	209mg

8. Blueberry Pancake

Preparation Time: *10 minutes* | ***Cooking Time:*** *20 minutes* |

Servings: *6*

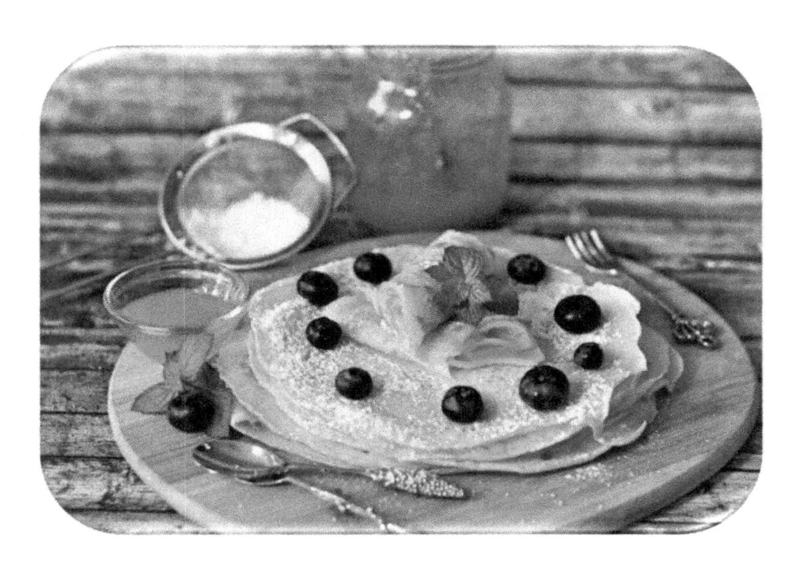

Ingredients:

- 2 tsp baking powder
- $1\frac{1}{2}$ cups plain all-purpose flour
- 1 cup buttermilk
- 3 tbsp sugar
- 2 eggs, slightly beaten
- 2 tbsp no-salt margarine, melted
- 1 cup canned blueberries, rinsed or 1 cup frozen, rinsed

Directions:

Sift together sugar, baking powder, and flour into a mixing bowl.

Make a well in the center, then add remaining ingredients. Mix into a smooth batter. Heat a heavy skillet or griddle, and grease it lightly.

Spooning out pancakes and cook until bottom is done. Flip and finish cooking.

Nutrition	Calories	Fat	Carbs	Protein	Sodium	Phosphorus	Potassium
	233	32g	7g	7.3g	91mg	29mg	109mg

Lunch Recipes

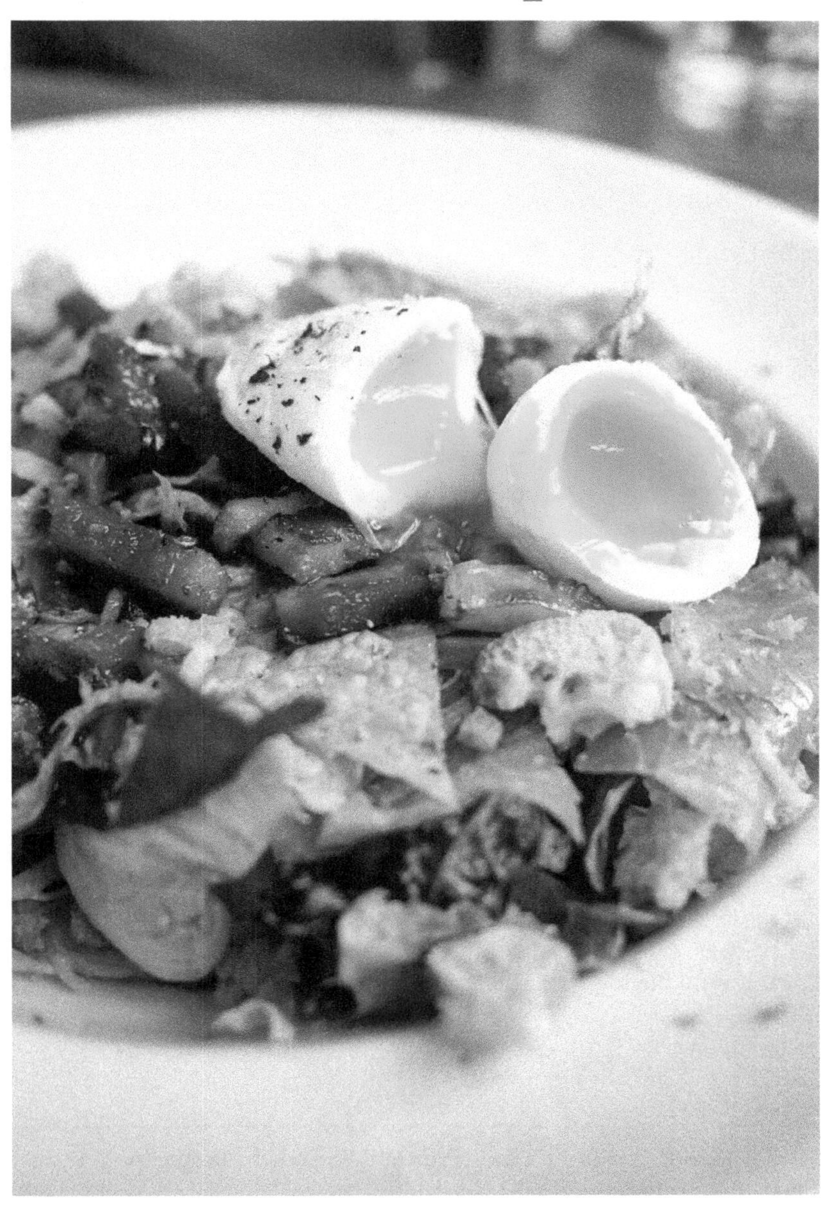

9. Green Pepper Slaw

Preparation Time: *5 minutes |* ***Cooking Time:*** *0 minutes |*

Servings: *12*

Ingredients:

- 2 medium carrots, peeled and chopped
- 1 small head of cabbage, chopped
- 1 medium green bell pepper, cored and chopped
- 2 teaspoons celery seed
- ½ cup Splenda granulated sugar
- ½ cup apple cider vinegar
- ½ cup water

Directions:

Take a salad bowl, place carrot, cabbage, and bell pepper in it and mix well until combined. Whisk together celery seeds, sugar, vinegar, and water until blended, drizzle it over the salad and toss until mixed. Serve straight away.

Nutrition	Calories	Fat	Carbs	Protein	Sodium	Phosphorus	Potassium
	76	0g	18g	1g	12mg	59mg	109mg

10. Easy Lemon Butter Salmon

Preparation Time: *5 minutes* | ***Cooking Time:*** *15 minutes* |

Servings: *5*

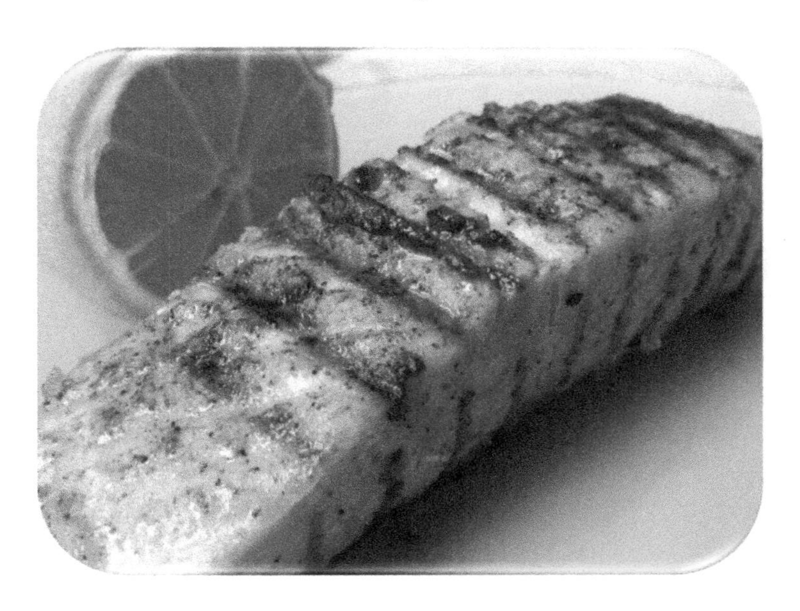

Ingredients:

- 2 tbsp minced garlic
- 1/2 cup butter, cubed
- 6 tbsp lemon juice
- 2 teaspoons salt
- 1/2 tbsp pepper
- 1/2 tbsp hot pepper sauce
- 5 salmon fillets or steaks

Directions:

In a small skillet, saute garlic in butter; whisk in lemon juice, salt, pepper and pepper sauce.

Transfer 2/3 cup to a serving bowl; set aside. Place salmon in a greased 15x10x1-in. baking pan.

Drizzle with remaining lemon butter. Broil 4-6 in. from heat 10-15 minutes or until fish flakes easily with a fork. Serve with reserved lemon butter.

Nutrition	Calories	Fat	Carbs	Protein	Sodium	Phosphorus	Potassium
	479	37g	2g	34g	117mg	59mg	209mg

11. Perfect Grilled Skirt Steak

Preparation Time*: 15 minutes* | ***Cooking Time****: 10 minutes* |

Servings*: 4-6*

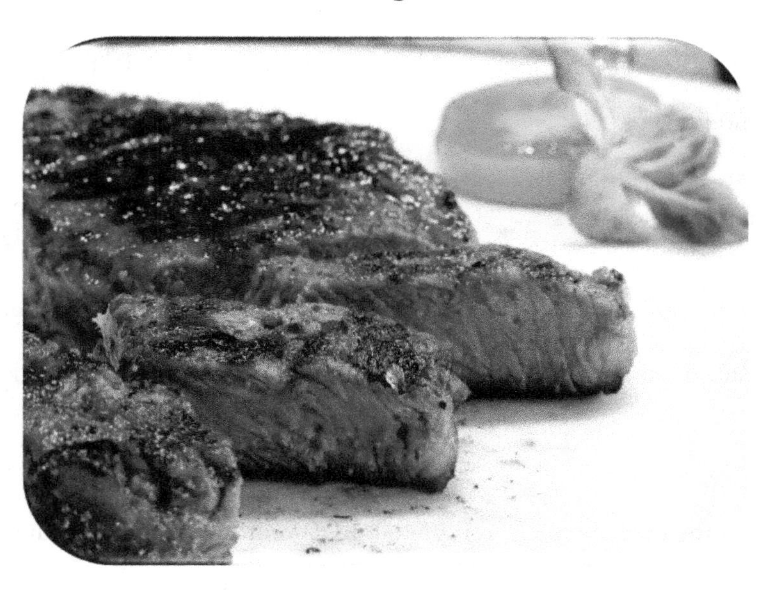

Ingredients:

- 1/4 cup canola oil
- 1/4 cup Meat Seasoning*
- 2 tbsp garlic, chopped
- 2 tbsp lemon juice, fresh
- 2 pounds skirt steak,
- Meat Seasoning
- Makes about 1/4 cup
- Ground black pepper
- 1 tbsp salt
- 1 tbsp ground cinnamon
- 1/2 tbsp paprika
- 1/2 tbsp dried thyme
- 1/2 tbsp granulated onion
- 1/2 tbsp granulated garlic
- 1/4 tbsp ground cumin

Directions:

In a small bowl, stir together the pepper, salt, cinnamon, paprika, thyme, onion powder, garlic powder, and cumin. Store the seasoning in a lidded glass container or zipped plastic bag in a cool, dark place for up to 1 month.

For the Steak:

In a small bowl, mix together the oil, seasoning, garlic, and lemon juice. Rub the mixture on both sides of the meat, making sure to work it into the meat.

Let the meat marinate at room temperature for at least 30 minutes but no longer than 45 minutes (if the day is very hot, don't leave the meat out for longer than 30 minutes).

Prepare a hot fire in a charcoal or gas grill and oil the grill grates. Grill the steak for 3 to 5 minutes on each side, until done to the degree of doneness you prefer. Let the skirt steaks rest for 5 minutes before slicing to serve.

Nutrition	**Calories**	**Fat**	**Carbs**	**Protein**	**Sodium**	**Phosphorus**	**Potassium**
	200	12g	3g	20g	190mg	65mg	310mg

12. Lamb Curry Stew with Artichoke Hearts

Preparation Time*: 10 minutes |* ***Cooking Time****: 1 hours and 20 minutes |* ***Servings****: 4*

Ingredients:

- ½ teaspoon black pepper
- ½ teaspoon curry powder
- ½ teaspoon ground cinnamon
- 1 clove garlic, minced
- 2 cups of beef broth
- 2 cups of water
- 2 tablespoons onion powder
- 1 tablespoon curry powder
- 1 tablespoon fresh lemon juice
- 1 tablespoon olive oil
- 1 teaspoon garam masala
- 1 teaspoon salt
- 1/3 cup manzanilla olives
- 14 ½ ounce fire roasted diced tomatoes
- 14-ounces artichoke hearts, quartered
- 2 teaspoon ginger root, grated
- 2-pounds lamb leg, trimmed from fat and cut into chunks

Directions:

In a bowl, combine the lamb meat with salt, pepper and ½ tablespoon of curry. Place a heavy bottomed pot on medium high fire and heat for 2 minutes.

Add oil and heat for 2 minutes. Add lamb meat and sauté until all sides are brown. Remove from the pot and set aside. Sauté garlic and ginger for a minute or two.

Pour the broth and scrape the sides or bottoms from the browning. Add the lamb back and place the rest of the ingredients except for the lemon juice.

Cover and bring to a boil. Boil for 10 minutes. Lower fire to a simmer and simmer until fork tender, around 60 minutes. Add the lemon juice and let it rest for 5 minutes before serving.

Nutrition	Calories	Fat	Carbs	Protein	Sodium	Phosphorus	Potassium
	436	18g	19g	7.5g	1471mg	259mg	1417mg

13. Beef Chow Mein in Zucchini Noodles

Preparation Time: *10 minutes |* ***Cooking Time:*** *1 hours and 20 minutes |* ***Servings:*** *4*

Ingredients:

- 2 zucchinis, processed into spaghetti-like noodles
- 1 egg omelet, julienned
- ¼ cup cilantro, minced
- For the Beef
- 2 teaspoons sugar and sea salt
- 1 tablespoon dark soy sauce
- 1 pound round steak, julienned
- For the Stir Fry
- 4 fresh shiitake mushrooms, caps julienned
- 4 leeks, sliced into inch-long slivers
- 2 tablespoons cornstarch, dissolved in 2 tbsp water
- 1½ tablespoons peanut or coconut oil
- 2 cups low-sodium vegetable stock
- 1-pound fresh bean sprouts
- 1 can bamboo shoot strip

Directions:

Place beef and marinade ingredients into a large food-safe bag; seal. Massage contents of bag to combine. Marinate in fridge for at least 30 minutes prior to use (or up to 42 hours before hand.) Drain well; reserve marinade for later.

Pour ½ tablespoon of oil into large nonstick wok set over medium heat; stir-fry zoodles until lightly seared. Transfer to plate lined with paper towels to remove excess moisture. Set aside.

Pour ½ tablespoon of oil into same wok. Cooking in batches, stir-fry half of marinated beef until brown on all sides; transfer to a plate. Repeat step for remaining beef.

Return beef to wok, along with beef stock, cornstarch slurry, reserved marinade, and mushrooms. Boil; continue cooking until mushrooms are fork-tender.

Except for garnishes, add remaining ingredients into wok, including zoodles. Stir-fry until bean sprouts wilt, about 20 seconds. Turn off heat.

Spoon equal portions of chow mein on a plate; garnish with cilantro and sliced egg, then serve.

Nutrition	Calories	Fat	Carbs	Protein	Sodium	Phosphorus	Potassium
	376	1.8g	2.1g	47.3g	543mg	59mg	209mg

14. Mint Pesto Zucchini Noodles

Preparation Time: *10 minutes* | ***Cooking Time:*** *15 minutes* |

Servings: *4*

Ingredients:

- 1/4 cup sliced almonds, toasted
- 1 cup mint leaves
- 1/4 cup fresh dill
- 1 clove of garlic, chopped
- 1/4 cup extra-virgin olive oil
- 1/4 cup grated Parmesan cheese
- 2 tbsp lemon juice
- Salt and pepper to taste
- 3 medium zucchini

Directions:

For the almonds:

Heat oven to 350°F. Place slivered almonds in a single layer on a baking sheet, and toast for 8 minutes, or until they have browned slightly and just become fragrant.

Remove the sheet from the oven and immediately place almonds on a plate or in a bowl.

For the mint pesto:

Add mint leaves, dill, and garlic to the bowl of a food processor and process until the herbs are finely broken up. Add olive oil, Parmesan, lemon juice, and salt and pepper and process until creamy.

For the zucchini noodles:

Slice the very ends off of three zucchini and spiralize using the fine spiralizer blade (or your blade of choice). Add the zucchini noodles to a large mixing bowl and pour in the pesto sauce.

Toss to combine. Top with additional Parmesan, dill, mint, and/or toasted almonds for serving.

Nutrition	Calories	Fat	Carbs	Protein	Sodium	Phosphorus	Potassium
	169	15g	6.5g	4.3g	150mg	129mg	319mg

15. Beef Shanghai Rolls

Preparation Time: *10 minutes |* ***Cooking Time:*** *1 hours and 20 minutes |* ***Servings:*** *4*

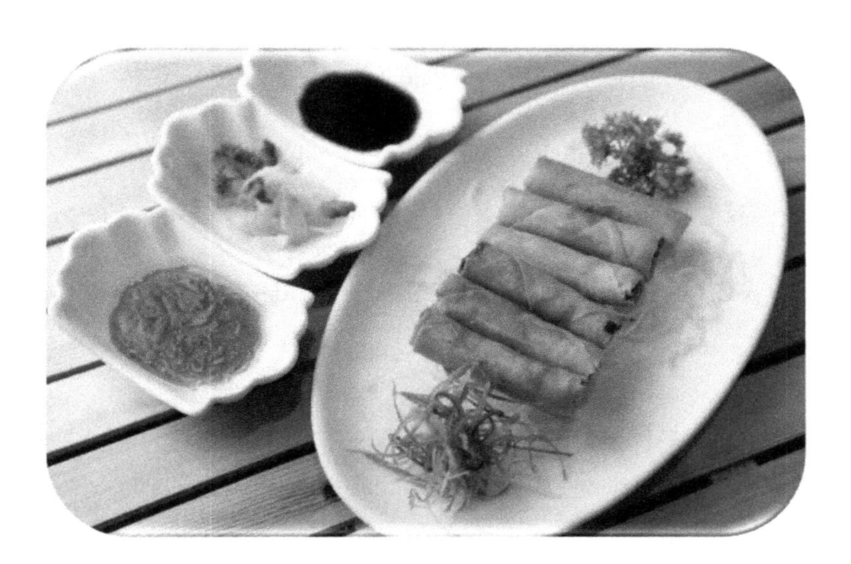

Ingredients:

- 4 tsp hot or sweet chili sauce, as dipping sauce
- 1 package rice paper wrapper,
- Water for sealing
- Oil for deep frying
- For the Filling
- 1 pound lean ground beef
- 1 shallot, minced
- 1 carrot, minced
- 1 garlic clove, grated
- 1 tsp low-sodium soy sauce
- 1 tablespoon fresh parsley, minced
- ½ cup butternut squash, minced
- ¼ cup fresh chives, minced
- ¼ cup sweet potato, minced
- Pinch of black pepper

Directions:

Mix filling ingredients in a bowl. Spoon 1 heaped tablespoon of filling in middle of spring roll wrapper; pinch and pull filling until you have a relatively straight but thin line that runs from one corner of wrapper to the other, leaving only an inch of space at the ends.

Dampen remaining edges with water. Fold wrapper over; start rolling tightly, leaving side edges open. Pinch edges; slice

off parts that don't contain any filling. Divide each spring roll in half. Repeat step for remaining fillings/wrappers.

Half fill deep fryer with oil; set at medium heat. When oil becomes slightly smoky, reduce heat to lowest setting; gently slide in spring rolls a few pieces at a time.

Cook for 15 minutes; wrapper should be light brown. (If it becomes too dark, your heat setting is too high. Turn down heat immediately.)

Transfer cooked pieces to a plate lined with paper towels. Place recommended number of pieces onto plates. Serve with hot or sweet chili sauce on the side.

Nutrition	Calories	Fat	Carbs	Protein	Sodium	Phosphorus	Potassium
	145	5g	2.1g	38g	285mg	59mg	605mg

16. Roasted Wedges of Cabbage

Preparation Time: *12 minutes* | ***Cooking Time:*** *35 minutes* |

Servings: *16*

Ingredients:

- 2 tsp sugar
- 1 green cabbage, cut into 1-in wedges
- 1 tbsp balsamic vinegar
- ¼ tsp freshly ground pepper
- 2 tbsp olive oil

Directions:

Preheat oven to 450°F, with baking pan heating inside, then combine sugar and pepper in a small bowl.

Brush cabbage wedges with oil. Sprinkle with pepper and sugar. Put the seasoned wedges on the hot baking sheet.

Roast until cabbage is browned and tender for 25 minutes. Drizzle with balsamic vinegar, then serve.

Nutrition	Calories	Fat	Carbs	Protein	Sodium	Phosphorus	Potassium
	323	2g	4g	0.5g	41mg	29mg	109mg

Dinner Recipes

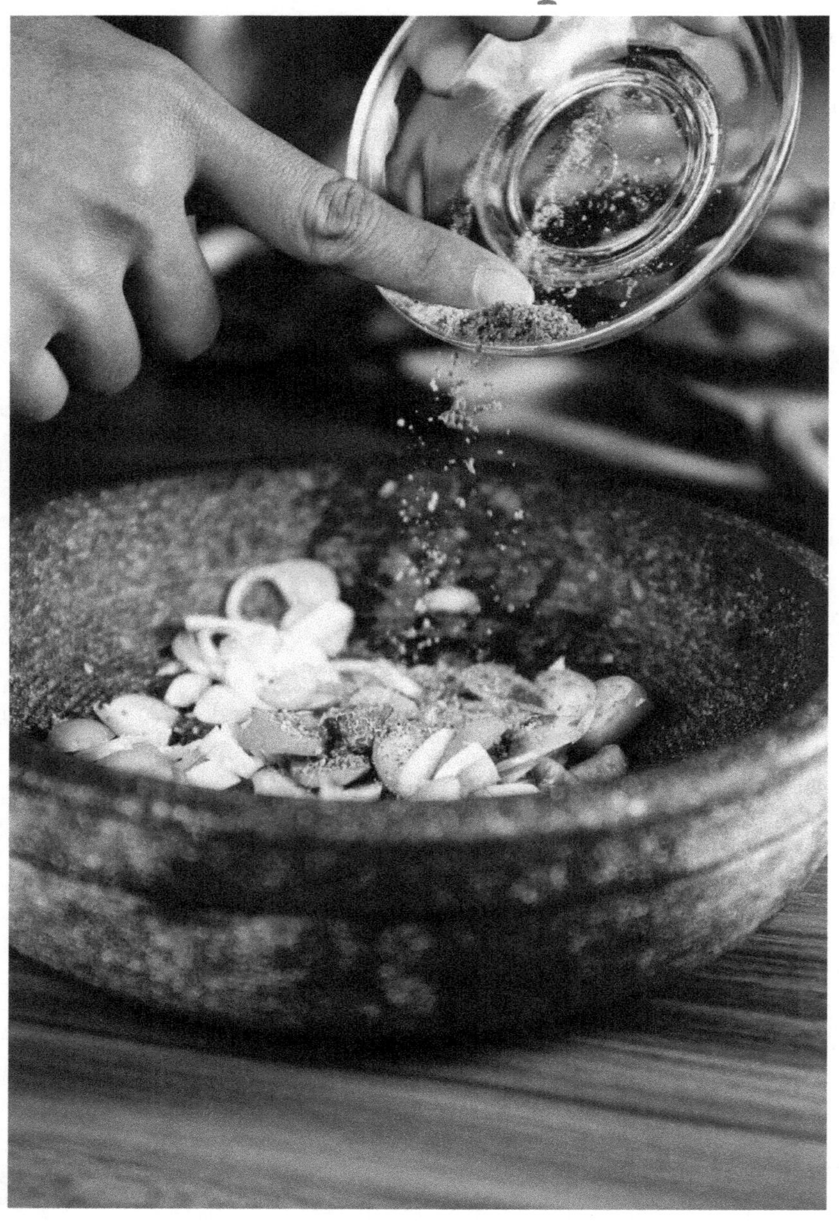

17. Steamed Bream with Fennel

***Preparation Time**: 10 minutes* | ***Cooking Time**: 20 minutes* |

***Servings**: 4*

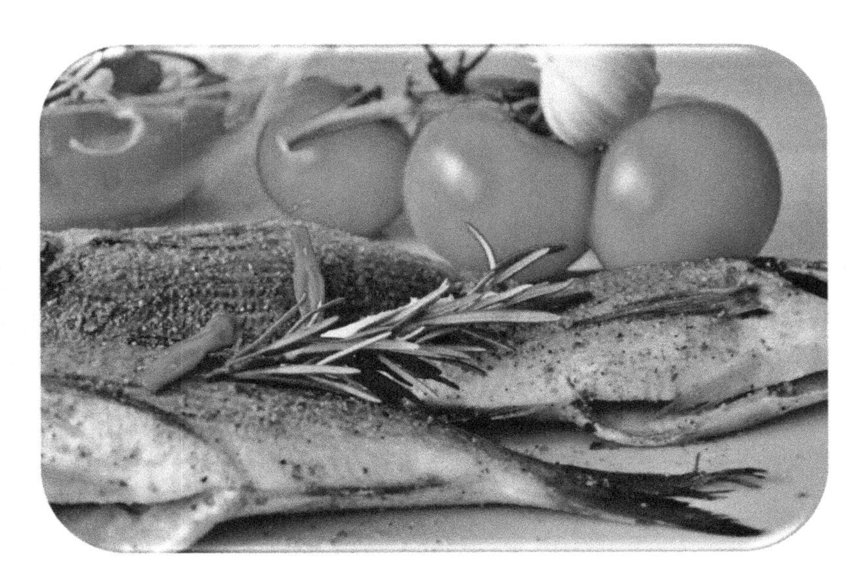

Ingredients:

- 2 Tbsp of olive oil
- 4 Tbsp of water
- 2 large spring onion, sliced
- 1 sprig of fresh rosemary, only the leaves, chopped
- 1 clove of garlic, crushed
- 4 fillets of sea bream (about 1 1/2 lbs.)
- Juice of 1 lemon
- 4 Tbsp of fresh fennel
- Salt and ground pepper

Directions:

Heat the olive oil in a large skillet. Add the spring onions, cover and cook for 7 - 8 minutes on medium heat.

Next, add the garlic, water rosemary, salt, pepper, stir and cook for 2 - 3 minutes. In a large pot heat water and set a steamer with the fish.

Cover the pot and steam the fish for 8 minutes.

Remove fish on a plate, and cover with the spring onion sauce. Sprinkle with chopped fennel, and drizzle with fresh lemon juice.

Nutrition	Calories	Fat	Carbs	Protein	Sodium	Phosphorus	Potassium
	281	12g	5g	38g	104mg	74mg	114mg

18. Egg and Fish Fry

***Preparation Time**: 15 minutes | **Cooking Time**: 15 minutes |*

***Servings**: 3*

Ingredients:

- 1 lbs. Fish fillet-skinless and boneless
- 1/2 Lime juice
- Sea salt
- 1 green onion
- 1/2-inch ginger
- 3 cloves garlic
- 1/2 cup cilantro
- 2 green chilies
- 1 egg
- 1 cup ground almonds
- Oil for frying

Directions:

Cut the fish fillet into pieces, rinse and pat dry. Put the fish fillets in a plastic bag and marinate with lime juice and the salt.

Make a fine paste with onion, ginger, garlic, green chilies and cilantro, using a food processor, Vitamix or blender.

Add the paste to the marinade and shake to combine well. Remove the fish pieces only, and discard the excess marinate.

Whisk the egg with 2-3 tbsp of water to have a smooth consistency.

Spread the ground almonds on a flat surface. Dip the fish piece in the egg mixture, and then roll into ground almonds.

Heat the oil in deep frying skillet. Fry the fish fillets until get a nice golden-brown color.

Remove from the skillet and place on a paper towel to absorb the excess oil, then serve very hot.

Nutrition	**Calories**	**Fat**	**Carbs**	**Protein**	**Sodium**	**Phosphorus**	**Potassium**
	125	6g	29g	15g	48mg	159mg	279mg

19. Tuna Salad with Avocado, Sesame and Mint

Preparation Time: *15 minutes* | ***Cooking Time:*** *15 minutes*|

Servings: *6*

Ingredients:

- 1 cucumber, sliced
- 1 pepper green, hot
- 1 avocado
- 1 zucchini, sliced
- Juice and zest of 2 limes
- 1/4 cup of olive oil
- Salt and ground pepper
- 1 lbs. of tuna, fresh
- 2 Tbsp of sesame seeds
- 2 - 3 Tbsp of fresh mint, finely chopped

Directions:

Cut the cucumber in the middle and then at 4 slices.

Clean and slice the pepper, avocado, zucchini and place in a large bowl. Pour with fresh lime juice and drizzle with olive oil.

Cut the tuna fish into large pieces, and season with the salt and pepper. Heat some oil in a skillet at high heat, and fry tuna slices for 2-3 minutes.

Remove the tuna from the pan and transfer in a salad bowl; gently stir. Sprinkle with sesame seeds and fresh mint and serve immediately.

Nutrition	Calories	Fat	Carbs	Protein	Sodium	Phosphorus	Potassium
	331	23g	9g	24g	235mg	255mg	147mg

20. Almond Breaded Crayfish with Herbs

Preparation Time: *20 minutes* | ***Cooking Time:*** *5 minutes* | ***Servings:*** *6*

Ingredients:

- 1 cup of grated almonds
- The zest of one orange
- 1 bunch of parsley
- 3/4 cup of olive oil
- Salt and ground pepper
- 30 crayfish, cleaned
- 2 lemons For serving

Directions:

Place grated almonds, orange zest, parsley, 3 tablespoons of oil, and the salt and ground pepper in a blender.

Pour the almond mixture to the deep plate and roll on each crayfish.

Heat the oil in a large skillet over high heat. Cook crayfish for 5 minutes turning 2 - 3 times. Serve hot with lemon wedges.

Nutrition	Calories	Fat	Carbs	Protein	Sodium	Phosphorus	Potassium
	489	9g	9g	12g	79mg	106mg	213mg

21. Aromatic Cuttlefish with Spinach

***Preparation Time**: 10 minutes* | ***Cooking Time**: 1 hour* |

***Servings**: 6*

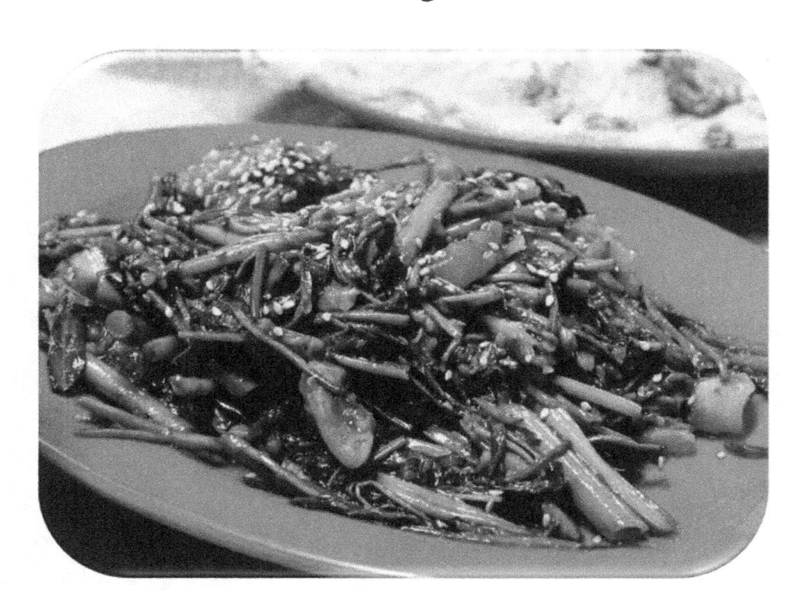

Ingredients:

- 2 lbs. of cuttlefish
- 3/4 cup of olive oil
- 3 cups of water
- 3/4 cup of fresh anis
- 1 lbs. of fresh spinach
- 1 small tomato, grated
- Juice of 1 large lemon
- Salt and pepper to taste

Directions:

Clean and rinse thoroughly the cuttlefish. Heat the oil in a large skillet and sauté the onion for 1-2 minutes over medium heat.

Add the cuttlefish and cook until get the color. Pour 3 cups of water, close the pot lid and simmer for at least 40-45 minutes.

Add the spinach, anis, grated tomato, salt and ground pepper.

Close the lid again and continue cooking at low temperature until the herbs soften.

Pour in the lemon juice and mix well, then serve warm.

Nutrition	Calories	Fat	Carbs	Protein	Sodium	Phosphorus	Potassium
	378	28g	5.5g	27g	109mg	253mg	292mg

22. Baked Shrimp Saganaki with Feta

Preparation Time: *10 minutes* | ***Cooking Time:*** *15 minutes* |

Servings: *6*

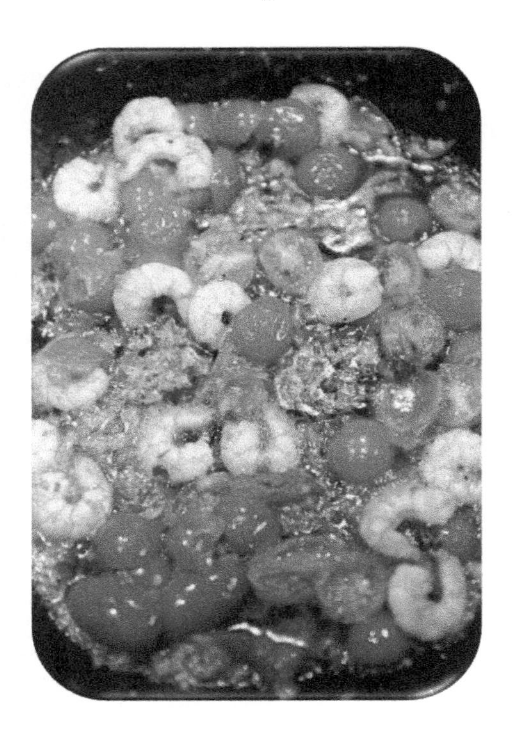

Ingredients:

- 1 cup of olive oil
- 1 large grated tomato
- 1 green onion, sliced
- 2 lbs. of large shrimp
- 2 cups of feta cheese, crumbled
- Salt and pepper to taste
- 1 cup of fresh parsley

Directions:

Preheat the oven to 350° F. In a large skillet heat the olive oil and cook the green onion and tomato.

Season with the salt and pepper and cook for 2 minutes, then add shrimp and stir for 2 minutes. Finally, sprinkle feta cheese evenly over the shrimp.

Place in oven and bake for 6 -8 minutes. Serve hot with chopped parsley.

Nutrition	Calories	Fat	Carbs	Protein	Sodium	Phosphorus	Potassium
	516	48g	5g	28g	174mg	172mg	192mg

23. Breaded Catfish Fillets

Preparation Time: *15 minutes |* ***Cooking Time:*** *10 minutes | **Servings:** 4*

Ingredients:

- 1/2 cup ground almonds
- 1/2 tsp sea salt
- 1/8 tsp freshly-ground black pepper
- 1/2 tsp of garlic powder
- 1 1/2 lbs. catfish fillets
- 2 eggs, beaten
- Olive oil for frying

Directions:

In a bowl, combine ground almonds, salt, garlic powder and pepper. Dip catfish fillets in beaten egg, then coat well with the almond mixture.

Heat the oil in a large skillet and cook breaded fish for 4 minutes from each side over medium heat. Turn only once during cooking and serve hot.

Nutrition	Calories	Fat	Carbs	Protein	Sodium	Phosphorus	Potassium
	410	29g	6g	32g	103mg	103mg	179mg

24. Calamari and Shrimp Stew

Preparation Time: *10 minutes* | ***Cooking Time:*** *15 minutes* | ***Servings:*** *4*

Ingredients:

- 3 Tbsp olive oil
- 1 green onion, finely chopped
- 3 cloves garlic, minced
- 3 lbs. shrimp cleaned and deveined
- 1 lbs. of calamari rings, frozen
- 1/4 can of white wine
- 1/2 can fresh parsley, finely chopped
- 1 grated tomato
- Salt and freshly ground black pepper

Directions:

Add the shrimps and calamari rings.

Stir and cook for about 3 - 4 minutes over medium heat. Add the wine, parsley and grated tomato.

Season the salt and pepper to taste. Cover and cook for 4 -5 minutes. Serve hot with chopped parsley.

Nutrition	Calories	Fat	Carbs	Protein	Sodium	Phosphorus	Potassium
	184	7g	4.5g	24g	87mg	201mg	192mg

Snacks & Sides Recipes

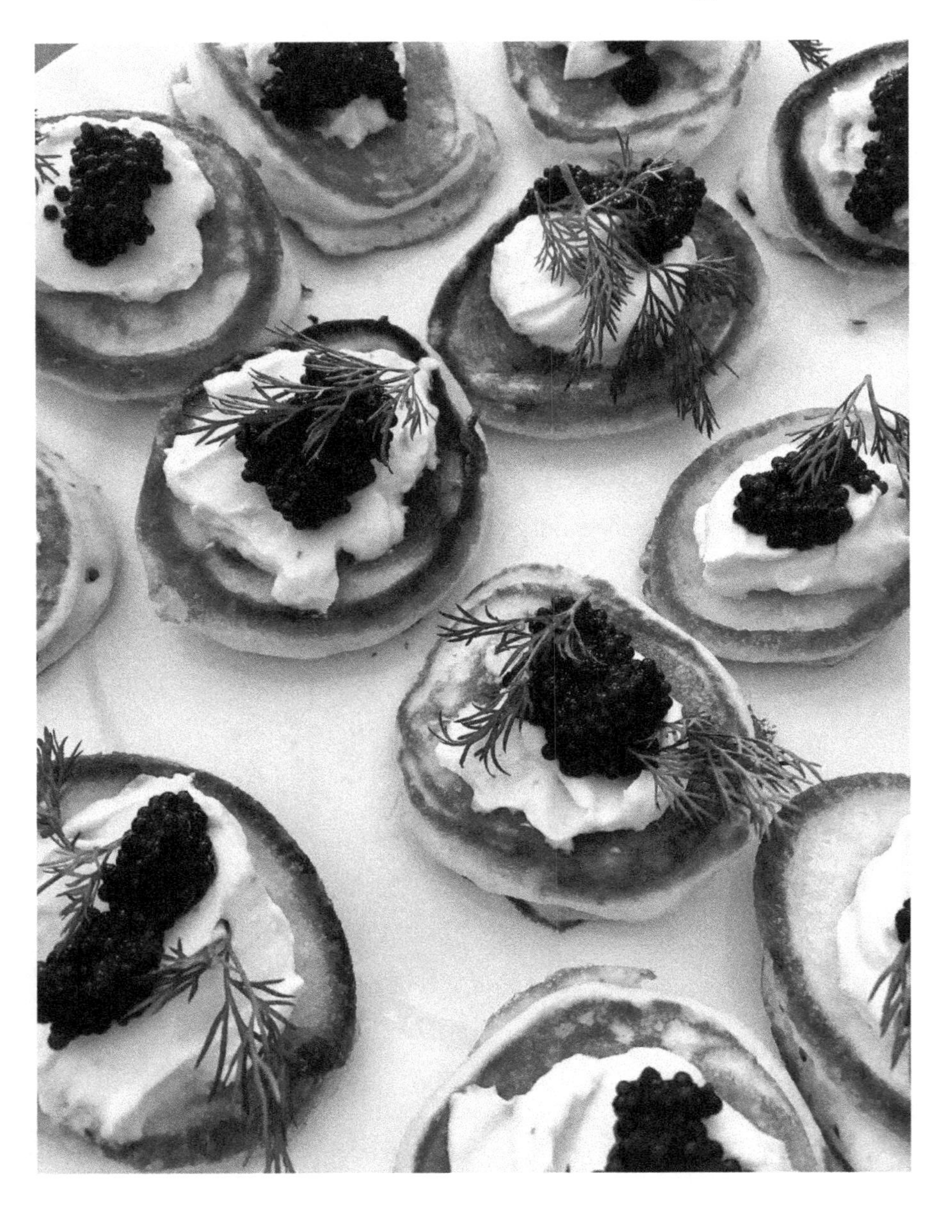

25. Fluffy Mock Pancakes

Preparation Time: *5 minutes* | ***Cooking Time:*** *10 minutes* |

Servings: *2*

Ingredients:

- 1 egg
- 1 cup ricotta cheese
- 1 teaspoon cinnamon
- 2 tablespoons honey, add more if needed

Directions:

Using a blender, put together egg, honey, cinnamon, and ricotta cheese. Process until all ingredients are well combined.

Pour an equal amount of the blended mixture into the pan. Cook each pancake for 4 minutes on both sides, then serve.

Nutrition	Calories	Fat	Carbs	Protein	Sodium	Phosphorus	Potassium
	188	15g	5.5g	9g	174mg	103mg	102mg

26. Mixes of Snack

Preparation Time: *10 minutes |* ***Cooking Time:*** *1 hours and 15 minutes |* ***Servings:*** *4*

Ingredients:

- 6 c. margarine
- 2 tbsp. Worcestershire sauce
- 1 ½ tbsp. spice salt
- ¾ c. garlic powder
- ½ tsp. onion powder
- 3 cups Crispix
- 3 cups Cheerios
- 3 cups corn flakes
- 1 cup Kix
- 1 cup pretzels
- 1 cup broken bagel chips into 1-inch pieces

Directions:

Preheat the oven to 250°F. Melt the margarine in a large roasting pan. Stir in the seasoning.

Gradually add the ingredients remaining by mixing so that the coating is uniform.

Cook 1 hour, stirring every 15 minutes. Spread on paper towels to let cool. Store in a tightly closed container.

Nutrition	Calories	Fat	Carbs	Protein	Sodium	Phosphorus	Potassium
	200	9g	27g	3g	3.5mg	47mg	110mg

27. Jalapeno Crisp

Preparation Time: *10 minutes* | ***Cooking Time***: *1 hour 15 minutes* | ***Servings***: *20*

Ingredients:

- 1 cup sesame seeds
- 1 cup sunflower seeds
- 1 cup flaxseeds
- ½ cup hulled hemp seeds
- 3 tablespoons Psyllium husk
- 1 teaspoon salt
- 1 teaspoon baking powder
- 2 cups of water

Direction:

Preheat your oven to 350 °F. Take your blender and add seeds, baking powder, salt, and Psyllium husk.

Blend well until a sand-like texture appears. Stir in water and mix until a batter forms.

Allow the batter to rest for 10 minutes until a dough-like thick mixture forms. Pour the dough onto a cookie sheet lined with parchment paper.

Spread it evenly, making sure that it has a thickness of ¼ inch thick all around. Bake for 75 minutes in your oven.

Remove and cut into 20 spices. Allow them to cool for 30 minutes and enjoy!

Nutrition	Calories	Fat	Carbs	Protein	Sodium	Phosphorus	Potassium
	156	13g	2g	5g	79mg	53mg	112mg

28. Raspberry Popsicle

Preparation Time: *2 hours* | ***Cooking Time:*** *15 minutes* | ***Servings:*** *2*

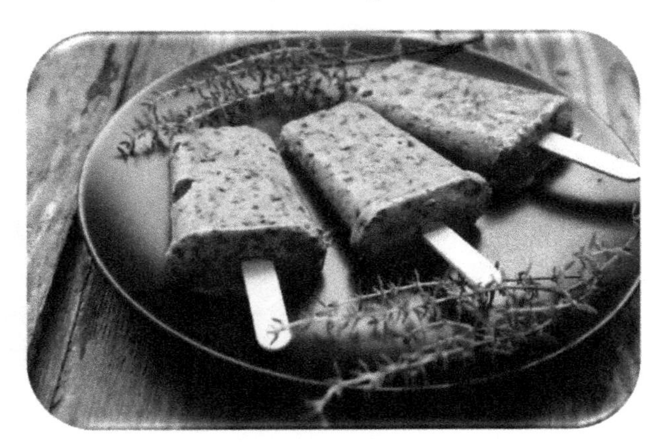

Ingredients:

- 1 ½ cups raspberries
- 2 cups of water

Direction:

Take a pan and fill it up with water. Add raspberries. Place it over medium heat and bring to water to a boil. Reduce the heat and simmer for 15 minutes.

Remove heat and pour the mix into Popsicle mold. Add a popsicle stick and let it chill for 2 hours. Serve and enjoy!

Nutrition	Calories	Fat	Carbs	Protein	Sodium	Phosphorus	Potassium
	58	0.4g	0g	1.5g	14mg	53mg	92mg

29. Easy Fudge

Preparation Time: *15 minutes + chill time |* ***Cooking Time:*** *5 minutes |* ***Servings:*** *25*

Ingredients:

- 1 ¾ cups of coconut butter
- 1 cup pumpkin puree
- 1 teaspoon ground cinnamon
- ¼ teaspoon ground nutmeg
- 1 tablespoon coconut oil

Direction:

Take an 8x8 inch square baking pan and line it with aluminum foil.

Take a spoon and scoop out the coconut butter into a heated pan and allow the butter to melt Keep stirring well and remove from the heat once fully melted.

Add spices and pumpkin and keep straining until you have a grain-like texture Add coconut oil and keep stirring to incorporate everything

Scoop the mixture into your baking pan and evenly distribute it.

Place wax paper on top of the mixture and press gently to straighten the top. Remove the paper and discard, then allow it to chill for 1-2 hours.

Once chilled, take it out and slice it up into pieces.

Nutrition	Calories	Fat	Carbs	Protein	Sodium	Phosphorus	Potassium
	120	10g	5g	1.5g	89mg	78mg	103mg

30. Cashew and Almond Butter

Preparation Time: *5 minutes* | ***Cooking Time:*** *0 minutes* |

Servings: *2*

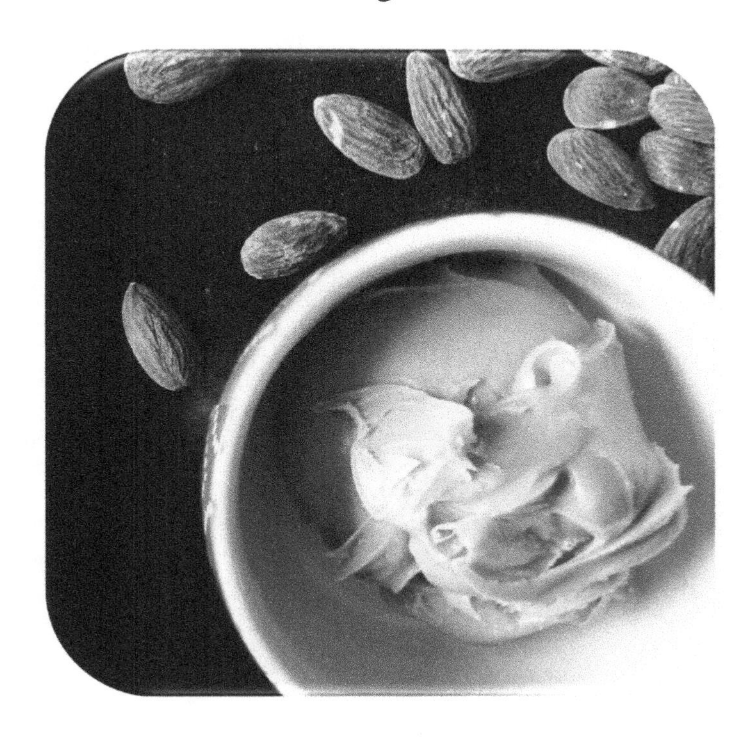

Ingredients:

- 1 cup almonds, blanched
- 1/3 cup cashew nuts
- 2 tablespoons coconut oil
- Salt as needed
- ½ teaspoon cinnamon

Direction:

Preheat your oven to 350 °F. Bake almonds and cashews for 12 minutes.

Let them cool Transfer to a food processor and add remaining ingredients

Add oil and keep blending until smooth Serve and enjoy!

Nutrition	Calories	Fat	Carbs	Protein	Sodium	Phosphorus	Potassium
	205	19g	9.5g	2.8g	107mg	79mg	152mg

Desserts Recipes

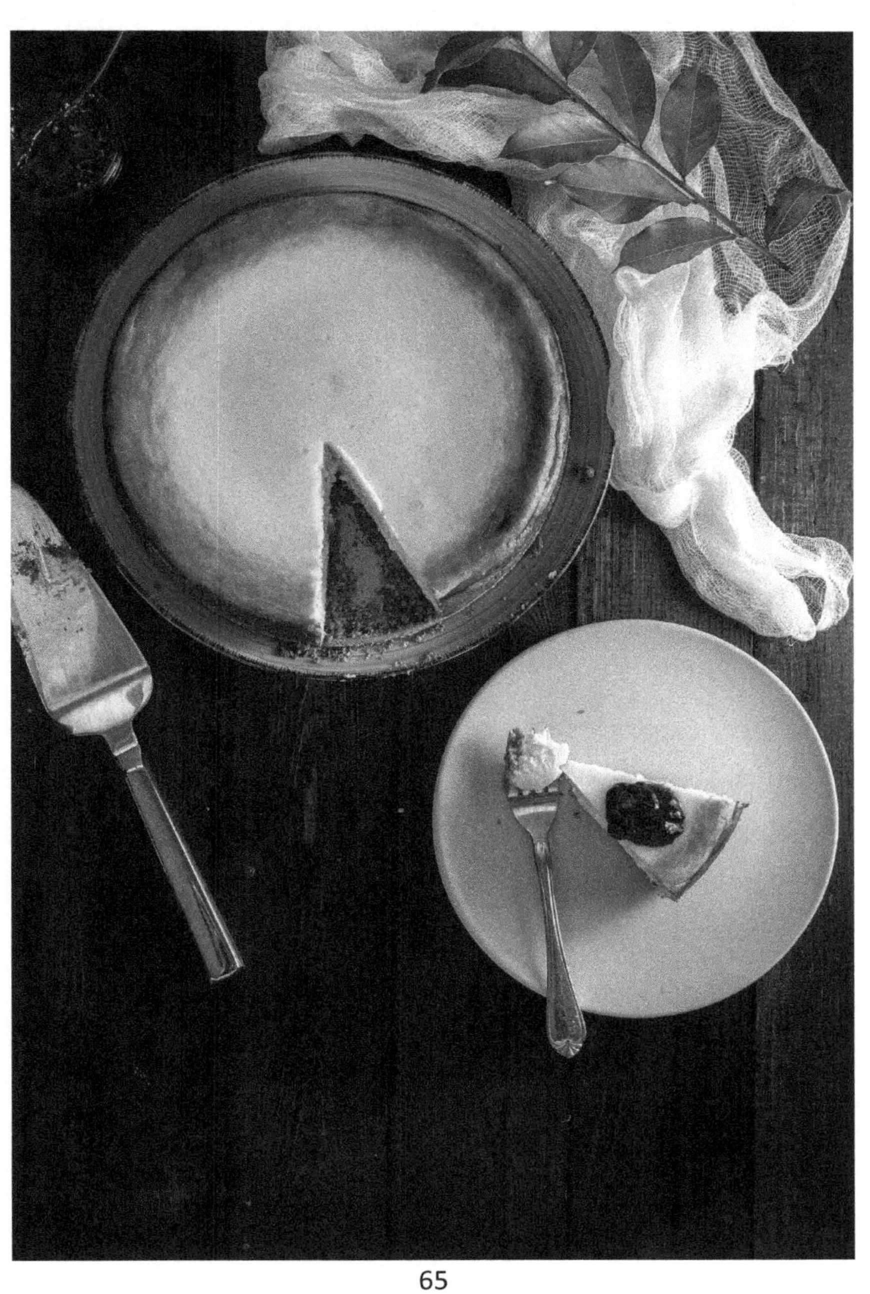

31. Date & Carrot Cake

***Preparation Time**: 10 minutes* | ***Cooking Time**: 50 minutes* | ***Servings**: 4*

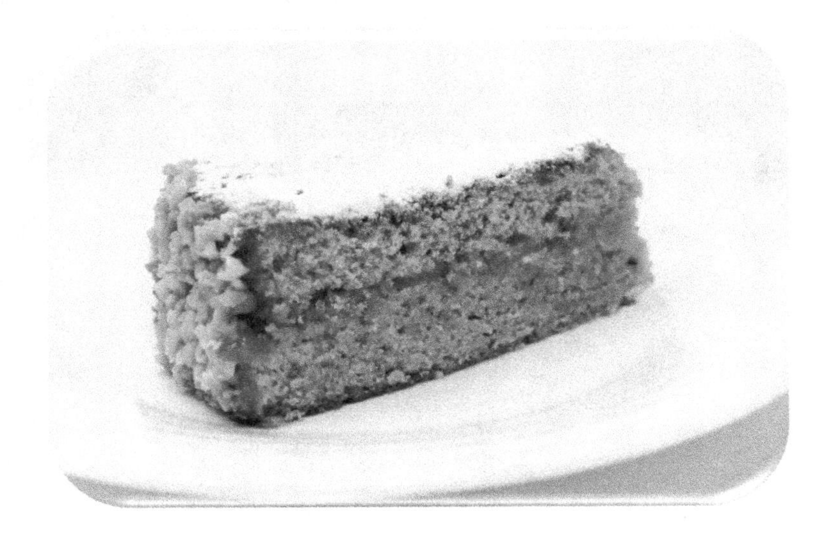

Ingredients:

- Dry Cake Ingredients:
- 2 cups whole wheat pastry flour
- 3/4 tbsp baking powder
- 3/4 tbsp baking soda
- 1/2 tbsp ground cinnamon
- 1/4 tbsp ground cardamom
- 1/4 tbsp ground allspice
- 1/4 tbsp ground ginger
- Wet Cake Ingredients:
- 2 tbsp ground flaxseed
- 1/2 cup almond milk
- 1/4 cup avocado
- 1/2 tbsp orange flower water
- Cake Mix in Ingredients:
- 1 cup shredded carrot
- 1 cup chopped dates
- Icing Ingredients:
- 1/2 cup cashews
- 1/2 cup chopped dates
- 1 cup water
- 1 tbsp orange flower water

Directions:

Start by adding 1.5 cups of water into Instant Pot and place a trivet over it. Grease a pan with cooking oil, suitable to fit the Instant Pot.

Prepare the batter by mixing the dry and wet Ingredients: separately. Now mix the two mixtures in a large bowl.

Spread this batter in the prepared pan then cover it with aluminum foil. Place the pan in the Instant Pot and seal its lid.

Cook for 50 minutes on Manual mode with high pressure.

Meanwhile prepare the icing by cooking cashews, date, and water in a saucepan to boil. Allow it to cool then blend this mixture in a blender until smooth.

Spread this icing over the baked cake. Slice and serve.

Nutrition	Calories	Fat	Carbs	Protein	Sodium	Phosphorus	Potassium
	184	9g	22g	4g	94mg	77mg	98mg

32. Pumpkin Chocolate Cake

Preparation Time: *10 minutes* | ***Cooking Time:*** *20 minutes* | ***Servings:*** *6*

Ingredients:

- 2 cups flour
- 1 tablespoon pumpkin pie spice
- 1 teaspoon baking soda
- 2 sticks- 1 cup unsalted butter, softened
- 1-1/4 cup sugar
- 1 egg
- 2 teaspoons vanilla extract
- 1 cup cream cheese
- 1 package 12 oz. chocolate chips

Directions:

Whisk pumpkin pie spice, flour and baking soda in a mixing bowl. Beat sugar with butter in a mixer until fluffy. Whisk in egg, vanilla, and cream cheese.

Beat well then gradually add the flour mixture while mixing continuously. Fold in the chocolate chips and grease 2 Bundt pans with cooking oil.

Divide the batter into the pans and cover them with aluminum foil. Pour 1.5 cups of water into the Instant Pot and place rack over it. Set one Bundt on the rack and seal the lid.

Cook for 20 minutes on Manual mode with High pressure. Once done, release the pressure completely then remove the lid.

Cook the other cake in the Bundt pan following the same method. Allow the cakes to cool then slice to serve.

Nutrition	Calories	Fat	Carbs	Protein	Sodium	Phosphorus	Potassium
	232	11g	30g	3g	112mg	46mg	103mg

33. Yummy Lemon Pie

Preparation Time: *25 minutes* | ***Cooking Time:*** *30 minutes* | ***Servings:*** *8*

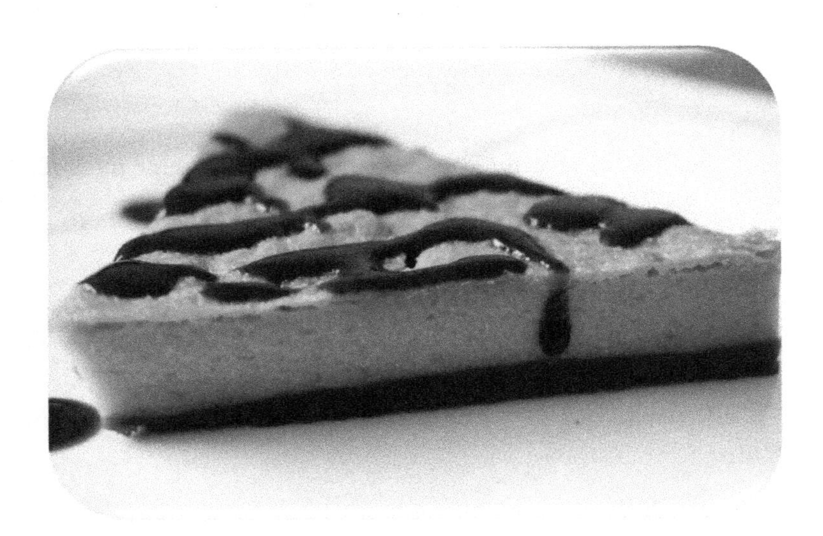

Ingredients:

- For the graham cracker crust:
- 1 and 1/2 cups graham cracker crumbs, 11-12 full sheets of graham crackers
- 1/3 cup granulated sugar
- 5 tbsp unsalted butter, melted and slightly cooled
- For the lemon pie filling:
- 1 cup fresh lemon juice
- 2 cans condensed milk
- 5 large egg yolks
- Topping:
- Whipped topping or homemade whipped cream

Directions:

To make the graham cracker crust:

Preheat oven to 350°F.

Combine the graham cracker crumbs and sugar in a mixing bowl and mix until well combined. Add the melted butter and stir until fully combined and all of the crumbs are moistened.

Scoop the mixture into a 9-9.5-inch pie plate and firmly press it down into an even layer on the bottom and up around the sides of the dish.

Bake at 350°F for 8-10 minutes or until the crust is lightly golden brown. Remove from the oven and set aside to cool for 5-10 minutes while you make the filling. Keep oven temperature at 350°F.

To make the lemon pie filling:

Combine the lemon juice, sweetened condensed milk, and egg yolks in a large mixing bowl and whisk until fully combined.

Pour the filling into the slightly cooled graham cracker crust and spread it around into one even layer. Bake at 350°F for 18-22 minutes or until the top of the pie is set, the pie will still be jiggly.

Remove from the oven and transfer to a wire rack to cool to room temperature for about 2 hours.

Transfer to the refrigerator to chill for at least 5-6 hours or overnight. Once chilled, top with whipped cream, serve and enjoy.

Nutrition	Calories	Fat	Carbs	Protein	Sodium	Phosphorus	Potassium
	362	16g	50g	5g	307mg	109mg	209mg

34. Tasty Gumdrop Cookies

Preparation Time: *10 minutes* | ***Cooking Time:*** *1 hour 30 minutes* | ***Servings:*** *4*

Ingredients:

- 3/4 cup shortening
- 1 cup sugar, divided
- 1/2 teaspoon almond extract
- 1-3/4 cups all-purpose flour
- 1/2 teaspoon baking soda
- 1/4 teaspoon salt
- 1 cup chopped fruit-flavored or spiced gumdrops
- 2 large egg whites

Directions:

Preheat oven to 350°F. Cream shortening and 3/4 cup sugar until light and fluffy.

Beat in almond extract. In another bowl, whisk flour, baking soda and salt; gradually add to creamed mixture and mix well. Stir in gumdrops.

In a separate bowl, beat egg whites until soft peaks form. Gradually add remaining sugar, beating until stiff peaks form.

Fold into dough. Drop by level tablespoonful's 2 in. apart onto ungreased baking sheets.

Bake until golden brown, 12-15 minutes. Cool 1 minute before removing from pans to wire racks to cool completely.

Nutrition	Calories	Fat	Carbs	Protein	Sodium	Phosphorus	Potassium
	102	4g	15g	1g	39mg	57mg	99mg

35. Almond Cookies

Preparation Time: *10 minutes* | ***Cooking Time***: *35 minutes* | ***Servings***: *24*

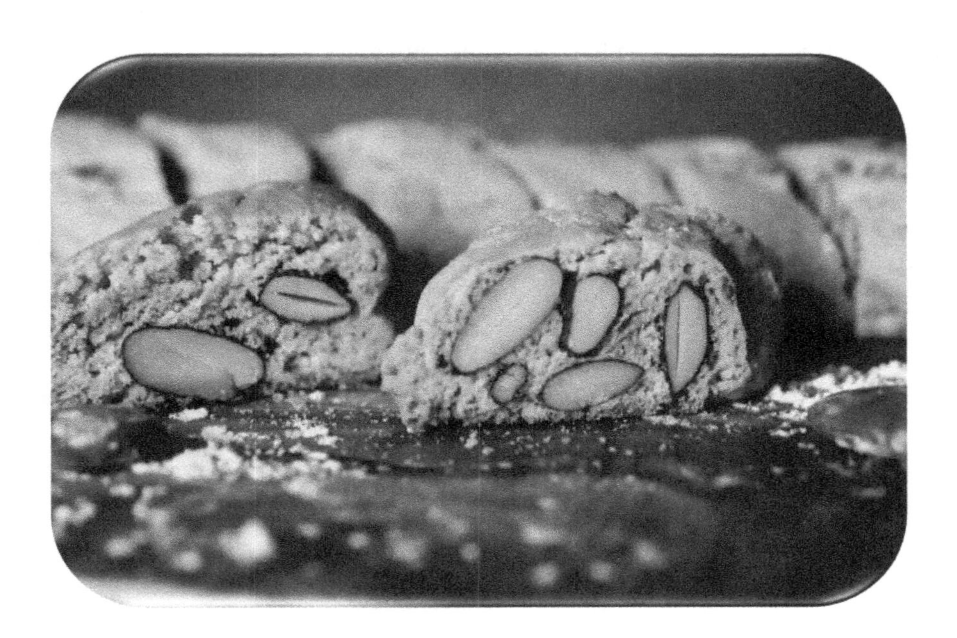

Ingredients:

- 1 tsp cream of tartar
- 2 egg whites
- ½ tsp vanilla extract
- ½ tsp almond extract
- ½ cup white sugar

Directions:

Preheat oven to 300°F. Beat egg whites with cream of tartar. Add remaining ingredients. Beat until firm peaks are formed.

Push one teaspoon full of meringue onto a parchment-lined cookie sheet with the back of the other spoon.

Bake for approximately 25 minutes or until meringues are crisp.

Nutrition	Calories	Fat	Carbs	Protein	Sodium	Phosphorus	Potassium
	184	9g	22g	4g	94mg	77mg	98mg

36. Blueberry and Apple Crisp

Preparation Time: *10 minutes* | ***Cooking Time:*** *25 minutes* | ***Servings:*** *8*

Ingredients:

- 4 tp cornstarch
- ½ cup brown sugar
- 2 cups grated or chopped apples
- 4 cups of fresh or frozen blueberries (not thawed)
- 1 tbsp lemon juice
- 1 tbsp margarine, melted
- ¼ cup brown sugar
- 1¼ cups quick cooking rolled oats
- 6 tbsp nonhydrogenated margarine, melted
- ¼ cup unbleached all-purpose flour

Directions:

Preheat the oven to 350°F. Combine the dry ingredients in the bowl.

Add butter, the stir until moistened. Set aside. Combine cornstarch and brown sugar, add lemon juice and fruits, then toss.

Top with crisp mixture. Bake for 1 hour until golden brown. Serve warm or cold.

Nutrition	Calories	Fat	Carbs	Protein	Sodium	Phosphorus	Potassium
	318	12g	52g	3.5g	114mg	201mg	244mg

37. Sweet Potato Brownies

Preparation Time: *5 minutes* | ***Cooking Time:*** *30 minutes*

| ***Servings:*** *6*

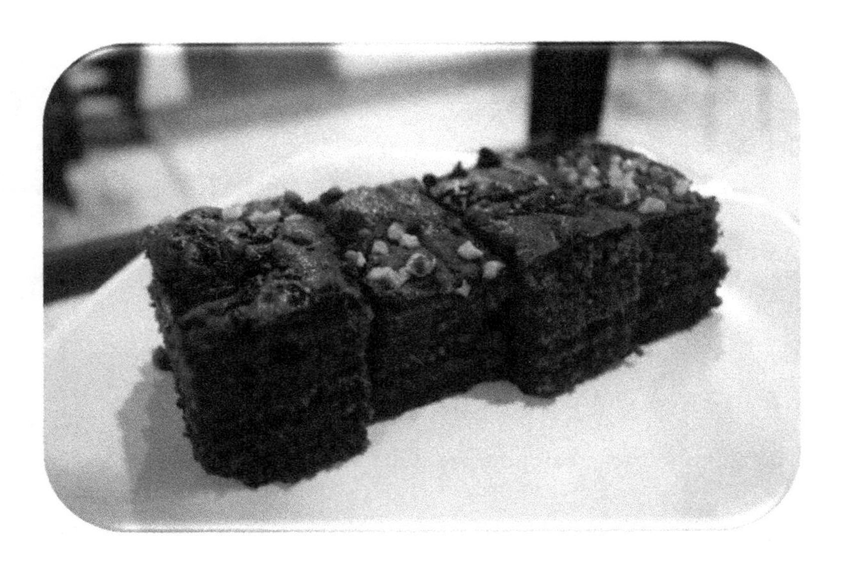

Ingredients:

- 1 tbsp cocoa powder
- 1 sweet potato, peeled, boiled
- ½ cup wheat flour
- 1 tbsp baking powder
- 1 tbsp butter
- 1 tbsp olive oil
- 2 tbsp Erythritol

Directions:

In the mixing bowl combine together all ingredients. Mix them well until you get a smooth batter.

After this, pour the brownie batter in the brownie mold and flatten it.

Bake it for 30 minutes at 365°F. After this, cut the brownies into the serving bars.

Nutrition	Calories	Fat	Carbs	Protein	Sodium	Phosphorus	Potassium
	95	4.5g	18g	2g	75mg	44mg	93mg

Smoothies & Drinks

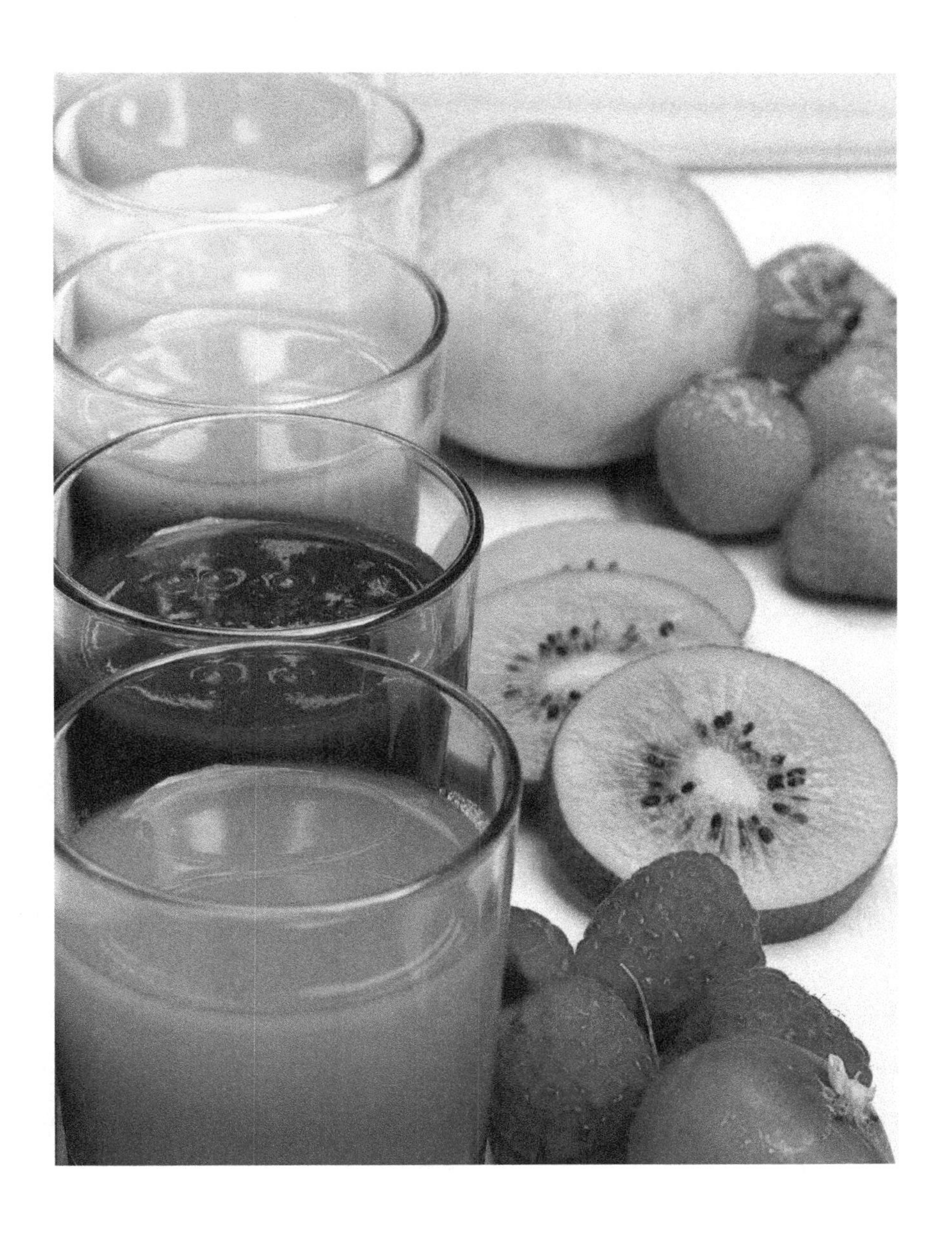

38. Apple and Beet Juice Mix

***Preparation Time**: 5 minutes* | ***Cooking Time**: 0 minutes* |

***Servings**: 2*

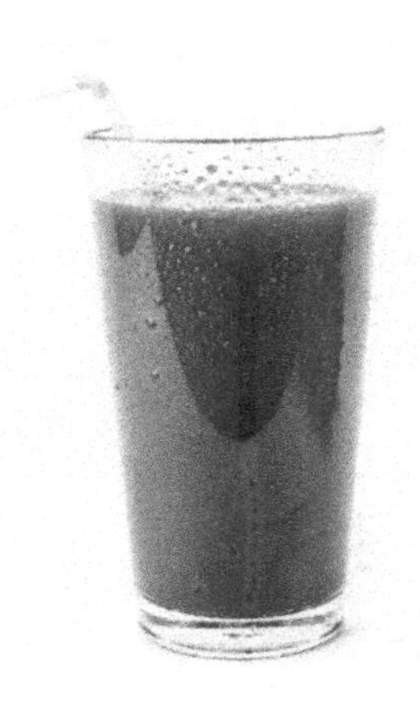

Ingredients:

- ½ medium beet
- ½ medium apple
- 1 celery stalk
- 1 medium fresh carrot
- ¼ cup parsley

Directions:

Juice all ingredients. Pour the mixture in 2 glasses and serve

Nutrition	Calories	Fat	Carbs	Protein	Sodium	Phosphorus	Potassium
	53	0g	13g	1g	12mg	41mg	13mg

39. Protein Caramel Latte

Preparation Time: *4 minutes* | ***Cooking Time:*** *10 minutes* |

Servings: *1*

Ingredients:

- 0,5 cups ounces of water
- 1 scoop whey protein powder
- 2 tbsp of Caramel Sugar-Free Syrup
- 6 ounces hot coffee

Directions:

Combine protein powder and water. Stir in coffee and caramel syrup.

Nutrition	Calories	Fat	Carbs	Protein	Sodium	Phosphorus	Potassium
	72	0g	1.3g	17g	19mg	19mg	103mg

40. Protein Peach Smoothie

***Preparation Time:** 4 minutes* | ***Cooking Time:** 0 minutes* | ***Servings:** 1*

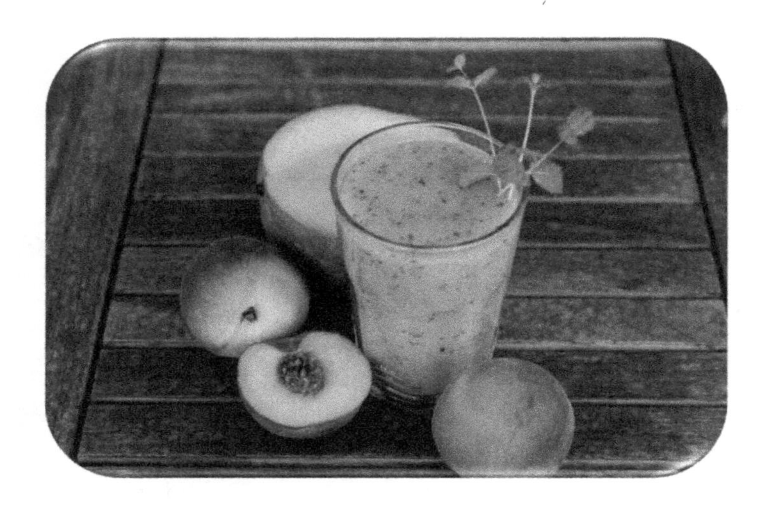

Ingredients:

- 1/2 cup ice
- 2 tablespoons egg whites, pasteurized
- 3/4 cup fresh peaches
- 1 teaspoon stevia

Directions:

First, begin by putting everything into a blender jug. Pulse it for 30 seconds until well blended. Serve chilled.

Nutrition	Calories	Fat	Carbs	Protein	Sodium	Phosphorus	Potassium
	195	0.2g	17g	24g	347mg	233mg	526mg

41. Cranberry Cucumber Smoothie

Preparation Time: *4 minutes* | ***Cooking Time:*** *0 minutes* | ***Servings:*** *1*

Ingredients:

- 1 cup frozen cranberries
- 1 medium cucumber, pe eled and sliced
- 1 stalk of celery
- 1 teaspoon lime juice

Directions

First, begin by putting everything into a blender jug. Pulse it for 30 seconds until well blended. Serve chilled.

Nutrition	Calories	Fat	Carbs	Protein	Sodium	Phosphorus	Potassium
	119	0.2g	25.1g	2.3g	21mg	185mg	325mg

42. Creamy Dandelion Greens and Celery Smoothie

Preparation Time: *4 minutes* | ***Cooking Time:*** *0 minutes* | ***Servings:*** *1*

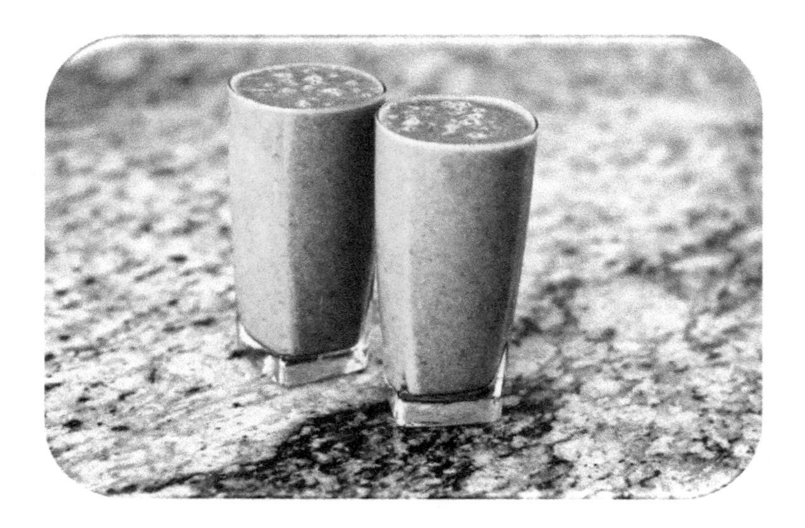

Ingredients:

- 1 handful of raw dandelion greens
- 2 celery sticks
- 2 Tbsp chia seeds
- 1 small piece of ginger, minced
- 1/2 cup almond milk
- 1/2 cup of water
- 1/2 cup plain yogurt

Directions:

Rinse and clean dandelion leaves from any dirt; add in a high-speed blender.

Clean the ginger; keep only inner part and cut in small slices; add in a blender. Add all remaining Ingredients and blend until smooth.

Serve and enjoy!

Nutrition	Calories	Fat	Carbs	Protein	Sodium	Phosphorus	Potassium
	58	6g	5.2g	3g	38mg	171mg	253mg

43. Dark Turnip Greens Smoothie

Preparation Time: *4 minutes* | ***Cooking Time***: *0 minutes* |

Servings: *1*

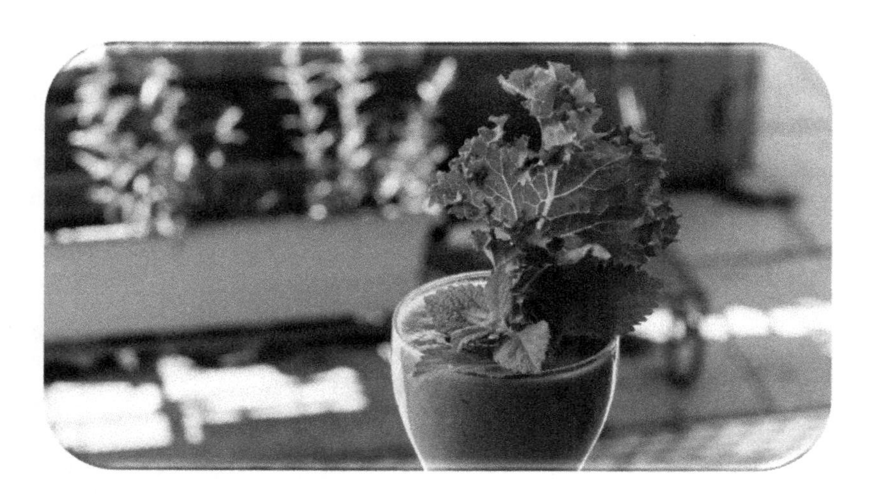

Ingredients:

- 1 cup of raw turnip greens
- 1 1/2 cup of almond milk
- 1 Tbsp of almond butter
- 1/2 cup of water
- 1/2 tsp of cocoa powder, unsweetened
- 1 Tbsp of dark chocolate chips
- 1/4 tsp of cinnamon
- A pinch of salt
- 1/2 cup of crushed ice

Directions:

Rinse and clean turnip greens from any dirt. Place the turnip greens in your blender along with all other Ingredients.

Blend it for 45 - 60 seconds or until done; smooth and creamy. Serve with or without crushed ice.

Nutrition	Calories	Fat	Carbs	Protein	Sodium	Phosphorus	Potassium
	131	10g	6g	6g	31mg	111mg	147mg

44. Butter Pecan and Coconut Smoothie

Preparation Time: *4 minutes* | ***Cooking Time:*** *0 minutes* |

Servings: *1*

Ingredients:

- 1 cup coconut milk, canned
- 1 scoop Butter Pecan powdered creamer
- 2 cups fresh spinach leaves, chopped
- 1/2 banana frozen or fresh
- 2 Tbsp stevia granulated sweetener to taste
- 1/2 cup water
- 1 cup ice cubes crushed

Directions:

Place Ingredients from the list above in your high-speed blender.

Blend for 35 - 50 seconds or until all Ingredients combined well.

Add less or more crushed ice. Drink and enjoy!

Nutrition	Calories	Fat	Carbs	Protein	Sodium	Phosphorus	Potassium
	268	26g	7g	6g	71mg	74mg	102mg

Salads

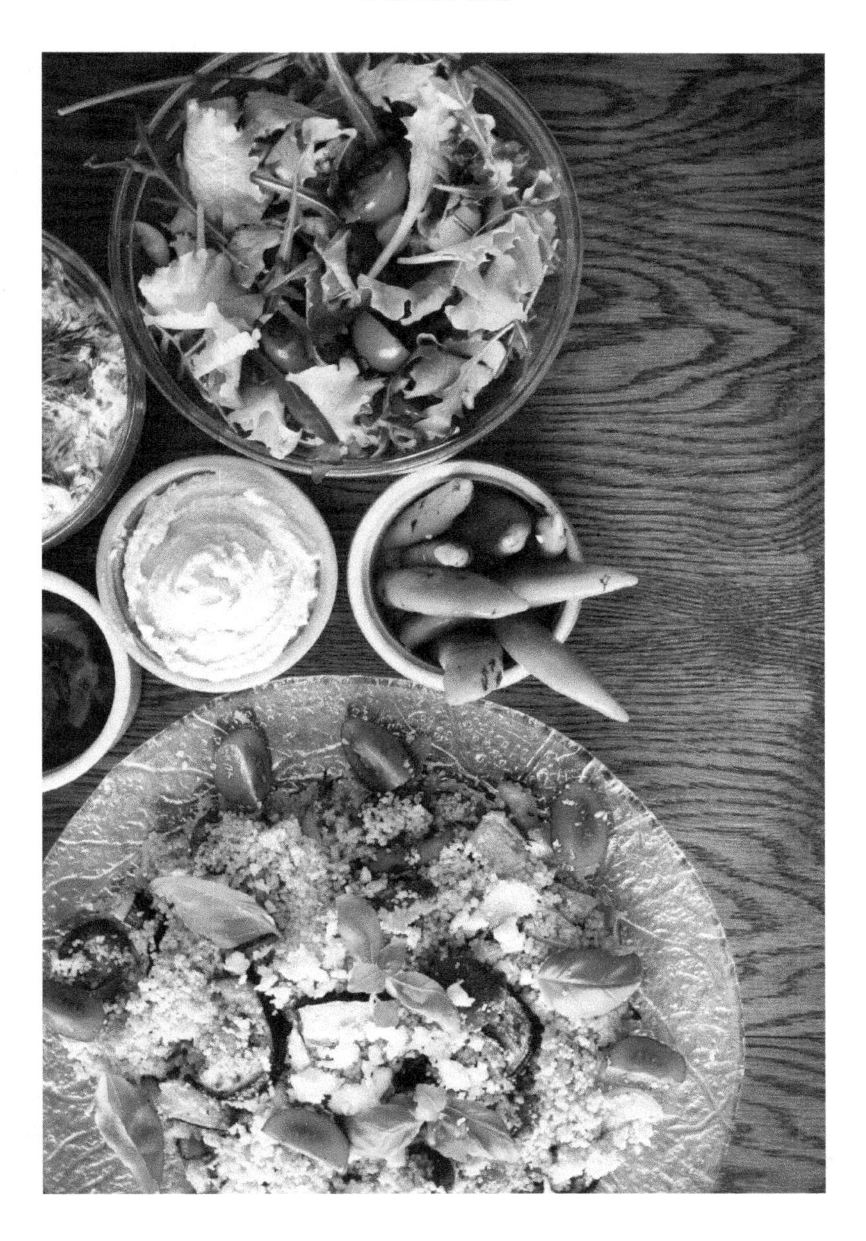

45. Lettuce, Asparagus and Raspberries Salad

Preparation Time: *25 minutes* | ***Cooking Time:*** *0 minutes* | ***Servings:*** *4*

Ingredients:

- Shredded green leaf lettuce – 2 cups
- Asparagus – 1 cup, cut into long ribbons with a peeler
- Scallion – 1, both green and white parts, sliced
- Raspberries – 1 cup
- Balsamic vinegar – 2 tbsp
- Ground black pepper to taste

Directions:

Arrange the lettuce evenly on 4 serving plates. Arrange the asparagus and scallion on top of the greens.

Place the raspberries on top of the salads, dividing the berries evenly. Drizzle the salads with balsamic vinegar. Before serving, season with pepper.

Nutrition	Calories	Fat	Carbs	Protein	Sodium	Phosphorus	Potassium
	36	0g	8g	2g	11mg	43mg	11mg

46. Waldorf Salad with Variation

Preparation Time: *20 minutes* | ***Cooking Time:*** *0 minutes* | ***Servings:*** *4*

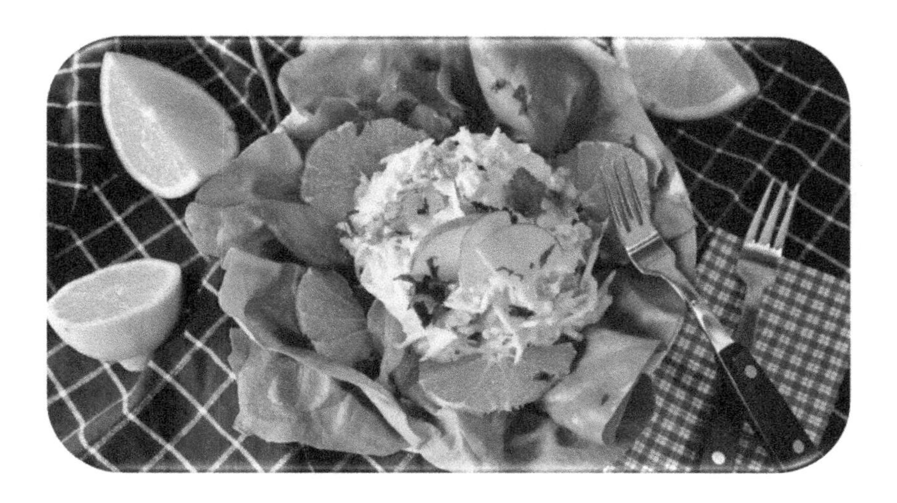

Ingredients:

- Green leaf lettuce - 3 cups, torn into pieces
- Halved grapes – 1 cup
- Celery stalks – 3, chopped
- Apple – 1, chopped
- Light sour cream – ½ cup
- Freshly squeezed lemon juice
- Granulated sugar – 1 tbsp

Directions:

Arrange the lettuce evenly on 4 plates. Set aside. In a bowl, stir together the grapes, celery, and apple.

In another bowl, stir together the sour cream, lemon juice, and sugar. Add the sour cream mixture to the grape mixture and stir to coat.

Spoon the dressed grape mixture onto each plate, dividing the mixture evenly.

Nutrition	Calories	Fat	Carbs	Protein	Sodium	Phosphorus	Potassium
	73	2g	15g	1g	30mg	29mg	193mg

47. Asian Pear Salad

***Preparation Time**: 30 minutes* | ***Cooking Time**: 0 minutes*

| ***Servings**: 6*

Ingredients:

- Shredded green cabbage – 2 cups
- Shredded red cabbage – 1 cup
- Scallions – 2, both green and white parts, chopped
- Celery stalks -2, chopped
- Asian pear - 1, cored and grated
- Red bell pepper – ½, boiled and chopped
- Chopped cilantro – ½ cup
- Olive oil – ¼ cup
- Juice of 1 lime
- Zest of 1 lime
- Granulated sugar – 1 tsp

Directions:

In a bowl, toss together the green and red cabbage, scallions, celery, pear, red pepper, and cilantro.

In a bowl, whisk together the olive oil, lime juice, lime zest, and sugar.

Add the dressing to the cabbage mixture and toss to coat. Chill for 1 hour and serve.

Nutrition	**Calories**	**Fat**	**Carbs**	**Protein**	**Sodium**	**Phosphorus**	**Potassium**
	105	9 g	6g	1g	48mg	17mg	136mg

48. Couscous Salad with Spicy Citrus Dressing

Preparation Time: *25 minutes* | ***Cooking Time:*** *0 minutes* |

Servings: *6*

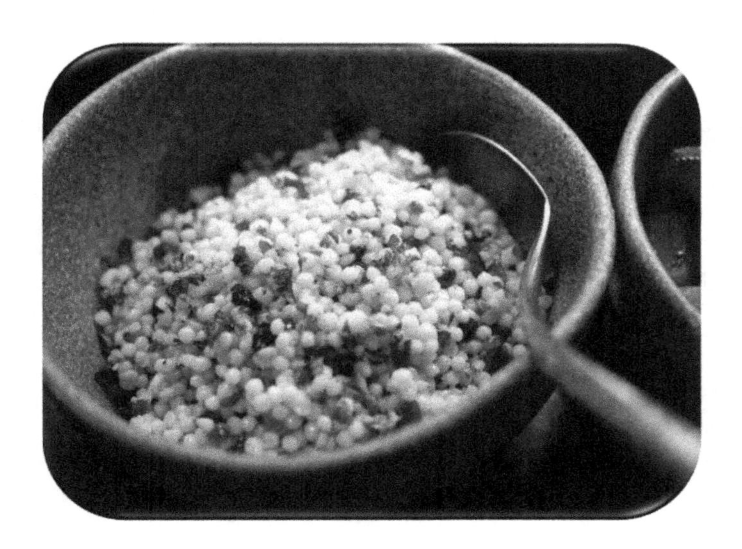

Ingredients:

- For the dressing
- Olive oil – ¼ cup
- Grapefruit juice – 3 tbsp.
- Juice of 1 lime
- Zest of 1 lime
- Chopped fresh parsley – 1 tbsp.
- Pinch cayenne pepper
- Ground black pepper
- For the salad
- Cooked couscous – 3 cups, chilled
- Red bell pepper – ½, chopped
- 1 Scallion, chopped
- 1 Apple, chopped

Directions:

To make the dressing, in a bowl, whisk together the grapefruit juice, olive oil, lime juice, lime zest, parsley, and cayenne pepper.

Season with black pepper.

To make the salad, in a bowl, mix the red pepper, chilled couscous, scallion, and apple.

Add the dressing to the couscous mixture and toss to combine. Chill in the refrigerator and serve.

Nutrition	Calories	Fat	Carbs	Protein	Sodium	Phosphorus	Potassium
	187	9g	23g	3g	5mg	24mg	108mg

49. Farfalle Confetti Salad

Preparation Time: *30 minutes* | ***Cooking Time:*** *0 minutes* |

Servings: *6*

Ingredients:

- Cooked farfalle pasta – 2 cups
- Boiled and finely chopped red bell pepper – ¼ cup
- Finely chopped cucumber – ¼ cup
- Grated carrot – ¼ cup
- Yellow bell pepper – 2 tbsp
- Scallion – ½, green part only, finely chopped
- Homemade mayonnaise – ½ cup
- Freshly squeezed lemon juice – 1 tbsp
- Chopped fresh parsley – 1 tsp
- Granulated sugar – ½ tsp
- Freshly ground black pepper

Directions:

In a bowl, toss together the pasta, red pepper, carrot, cucumber, yellow pepper, and scallion.

In a bowl, whisk together the mayonnaise, parsley, lemon juice, and sugar.

Add the dressing to the pasta mixture and stir to combine, then season with pepper. Chill for 1 hour and serve.

Nutrition	Calories	Fat	Carbs	Protein	Sodium	Phosphorus	Potassium
	119	3g	20g	4g	16mg	51mg	82mg

50. Tarragon and Pepper Pasta Salad

Preparation Time: *10 minutes* | ***Cooking Time:*** *35 minutes*

| ***Servings:*** *4*

Ingredients:

- Cooked pasta – 2 cups
- Red bell pepper – 1, finely diced
- Cucumber – ½, finely diced
- Red onion – ¼, finely diced
- Black pepper – 1 tsp
- Extra virgin olive oil – 2 tbsp
- Dried tarragon – 1 tbsp

Directions:

Cook pasta according to package

Cool and combine the rest of the raw Ingredients: and mix well. Serve.

Nutrition	Calories	Fat	Carbs	Protein	Sodium	Phosphorus	Potassium
	157	8g	24g	4g	5mg	61mg	92mg

Conclusion

You likely had little knowledge about your kidneys before. You probably didn't know how you could take steps to improve your kidney health and decrease the risk of developing kidney failure. However, through reading this

book, you now understand the power of the human kidney, as well as the prognosis of chronic kidney disease. While over thirty-million Americans are being affected by kidney disease, you can now take steps to be one of the people who is actively working to promote your kidney health. Kidney disease now ranks as the 18th deadliest condition in the world. In the United States alone, it is reported that over 600,000 Americans succumb to kidney failure.

These stats are alarming, which is why, it is necessary to take proper care of your kidneys, starting with a kidney-friendly diet. These recipes are ideal whether you have been diagnosed with a kidney problem or you want to prevent any kidney issue. With regards to your wellbeing and health, it's a smart thought to see your doctor as frequently as conceivable to ensure you don't run into preventable issues that you needn't get.

The kidneys are your body's toxin channel (just like the liver), cleaning the blood of remote substances and toxins that are discharged from things like preservatives in food & other toxins. At the point when you eat flippantly and fill your body with toxins, either from nourishment, drinks (liquor or alcohol for instance) or even from the air you inhale (free radicals are in the sun and move through your skin, through messy air, and numerous food sources contain them). Your body additionally will in general convert numerous things that appear to be benign until your body's organs convert them into things like formaldehyde because of a synthetic response and transforming phase.

One case of this is a large portion of those diet sugars utilized in diet soft drinks for instance, Aspartame transforms into Formaldehyde in the body. These toxins must be expelled, or they can prompt ailment, renal (kidney) failure, malignant growth, & various other painful problems.

This isn't a condition that occurs without any forethought it is a dynamic issue and in that it very well may be both found early and treated, diet changed, and settling what is causing the issue is conceivable.

It's conceivable to have partial renal failure yet, as a rule; it requires some time (or downright awful diet for a short time) to arrive at absolute renal failure. You would prefer not to reach total renal failure since this will require standard dialysis treatments to save your life. Dialysis treatments explicitly clean the blood of waste and toxins in the blood utilizing a machine in light of the fact that your body can no longer carry out the responsibility. Without treatments, you could die a very painful death. Renal failure can be the consequence of long-haul diabetes, hypertension, unreliable diet, and can stem from other health concerns. A renal diet is tied in with directing the intake of protein and phosphorus in your eating routine. Restricting your sodium intake is likewise significant. By controlling these two variables you can control the vast majority of the toxins/waste made by your body and thus this enables your kidney to 100% function. In the event that you get this early enough and truly moderate your diets with extraordinary consideration, you could avert all-out renal failure. In the event that you get this early, you can take out the issue completely.

CPSIA information can be obtained
at www.ICGtesting.com
Printed in the USA
BVHW062104250221
601128BV00006BA/485